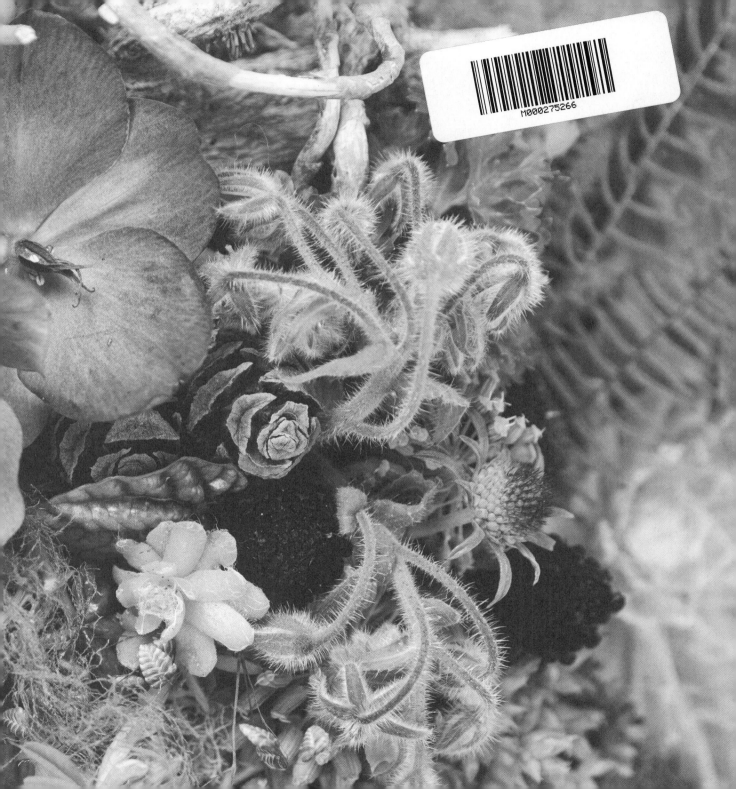

THE *Herbal* RECIPE KEEPER

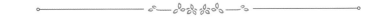

MY COLLECTION *of* HEALING PLANT REMEDIES *and* ESSENTIAL OIL BLENDS

WITH HERBAL ARRANGEMENTS BY FRANÇOISE WEEKS

PHOTOGRAPHS BY THERESA BEAR

Timber Press · Portland, Oregon

Published in 2018 by Timber Press, Inc.

The Haseltine Building
133 S.W. Second Avenue, Suite 450
Portland, Oregon 97204-3527
timberpress.com

Printed in China

Book design by Mia Johnson

ISBN 978-1-60469-887-9

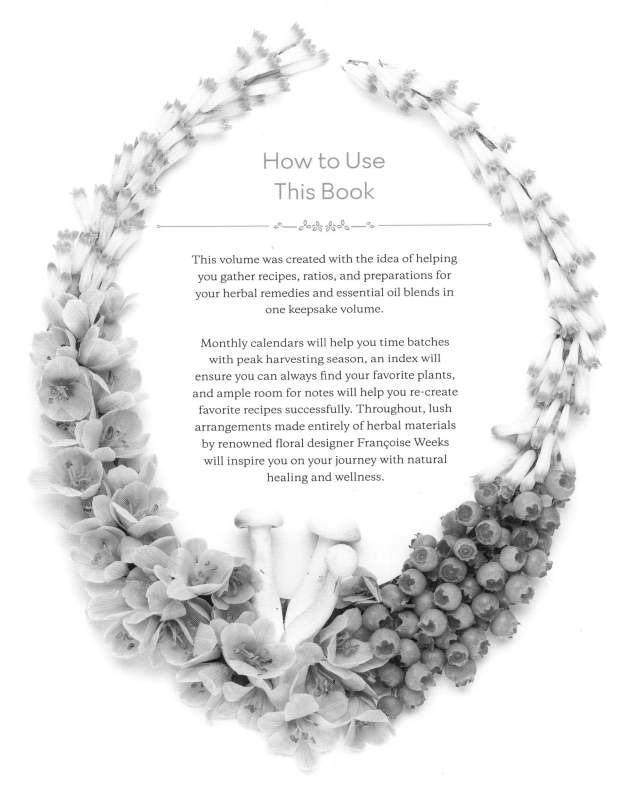

How to Use
This Book

This volume was created with the idea of helping you gather recipes, ratios, and preparations for your herbal remedies and essential oil blends in one keepsake volume.

Monthly calendars will help you time batches with peak harvesting season, an index will ensure you can always find your favorite plants, and ample room for notes will help you re-create favorite recipes successfully. Throughout, lush arrangements made entirely of herbal materials by renowned floral designer Françoise Weeks will inspire you on your journey with natural healing and wellness.

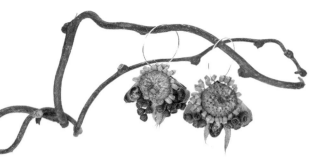

INDEX

Plant	Page		Plant	Page

Plant	Page		Plant	Page

Plant	Page		Plant	Page

Plant	Page

Plant	Page

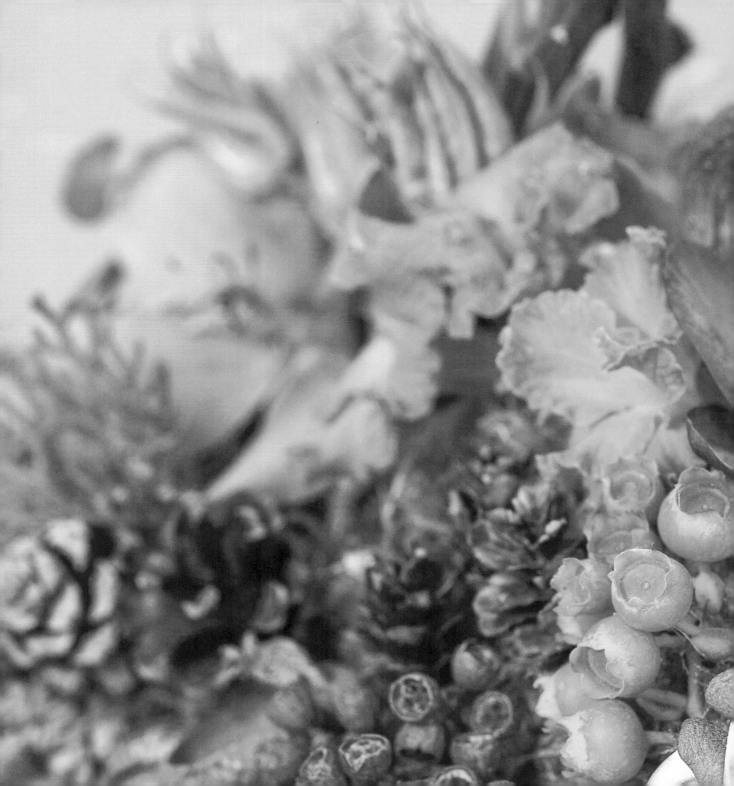

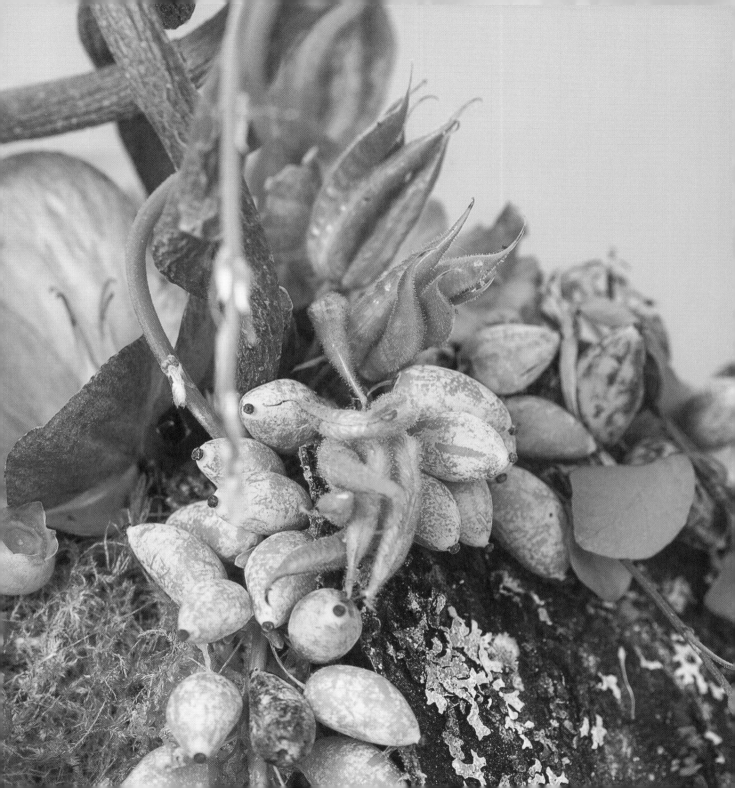

COMMON NAME

_____

BOTANICAL NAME

DATE

Parts used

Notes on the plant or harvest

Recipes or medicines created

Blends created with this herb's essential oil

Other preparations

10

_____

COMMON NAME

_____   _____

BOTANICAL NAME   DATE

Parts used

_____
_____
_____
_____

Notes on the plant or harvest

_____
_____
_____
_____

Recipes or medicines created

_____
_____
_____
_____
_____
_____
_____
_____
_____
_____

Blends created with this herb's essential oil

Other preparations

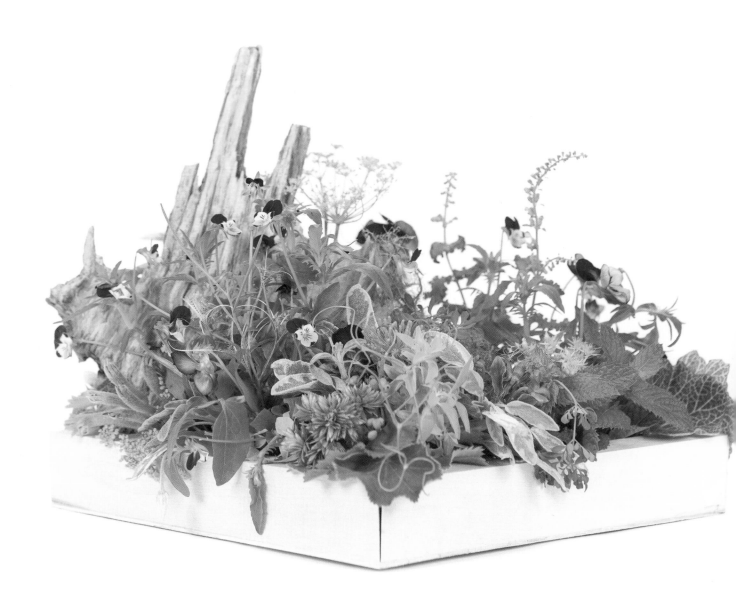

COMMON NAME

BOTANICAL NAME

DATE

Parts used

_____
_____
_____
_____

Notes on the plant or harvest

_____
_____
_____
_____

Recipes or medicines created

_____
_____
_____
_____
_____
_____
_____
_____
_____

Blends created with this herb's essential oil

Other preparations

COMMON NAME

BOTANICAL NAME

DATE

Parts used

Notes on the plant or harvest

Recipes or medicines created

Blends created with this herb's essential oil

Other preparations

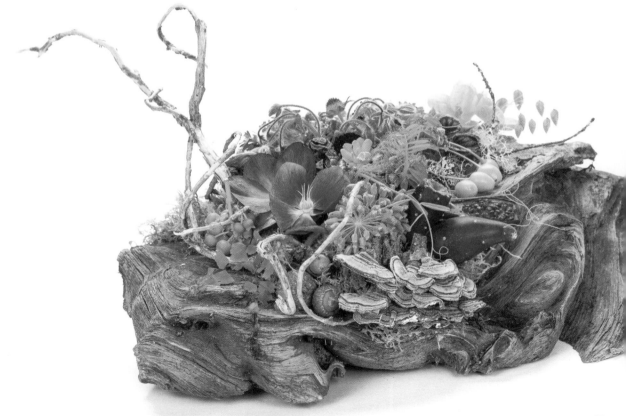

_____

COMMON NAME

_____   _____

BOTANICAL NAME   DATE

Parts used

_____
_____
_____
_____

Notes on the plant or harvest

_____
_____
_____
_____

Recipes or medicines created

_____
_____
_____
_____
_____
_____
_____
_____
_____

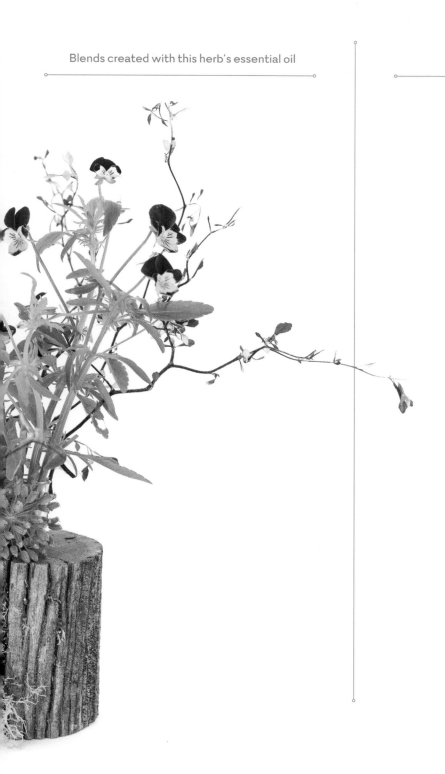

Blends created with this herb's essential oil

Other preparations

17

COMMON NAME

BOTANICAL NAME

DATE

Parts used

Notes on the plant or harvest

Recipes or medicines created

Blends created with this herb's essential oil

Other preparations

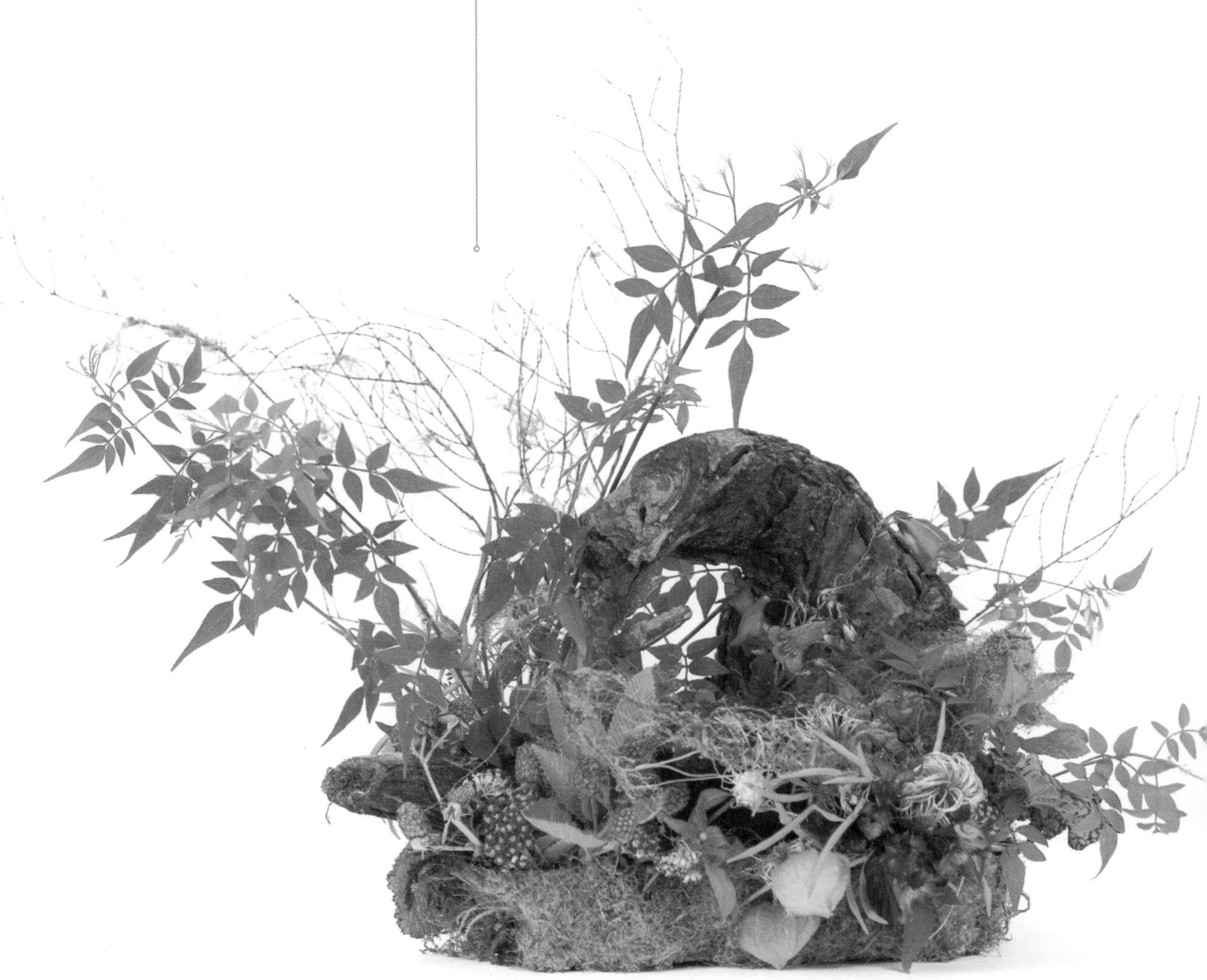

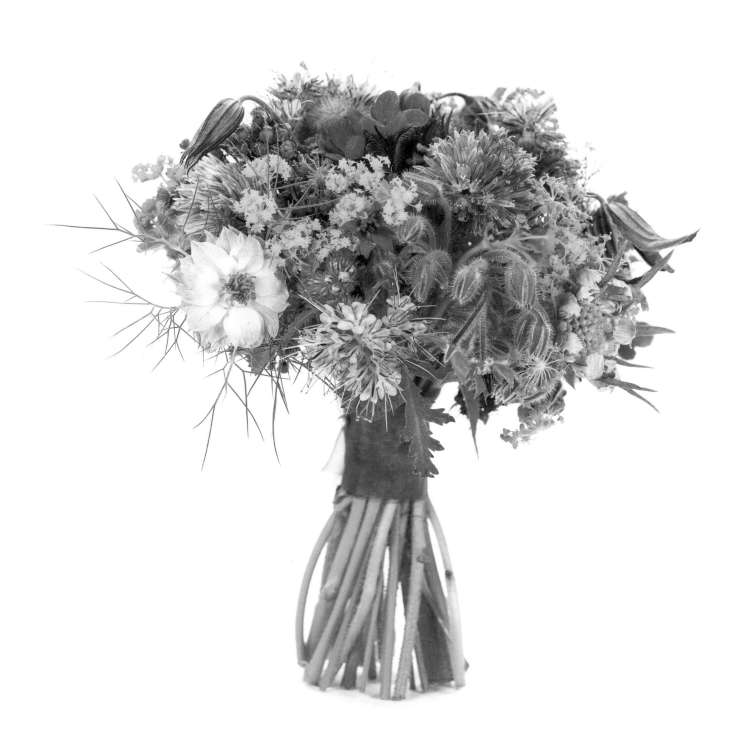

_____

COMMON NAME

_____   _____

BOTANICAL NAME   DATE

— ❧ ·❀·❀·❀· ❧ —

Parts used

_____
_____
_____
_____

Notes on the plant or harvest

_____
_____
_____
_____

Recipes or medicines created

_____
_____
_____
_____
_____
_____
_____
_____
_____

Blends created with this herb's essential oil

Other preparations

_____

COMMON NAME

_____

BOTANICAL NAME   DATE

———— ⚘⚘⚘⚘ ————

Parts used   Notes on the plant or harvest

_____   _____
_____   _____
_____   _____
_____   _____

Recipes or medicines created

_____
_____
_____
_____
_____
_____
_____
_____
_____
_____

Blends created with this herb's essential oil

Other preparations

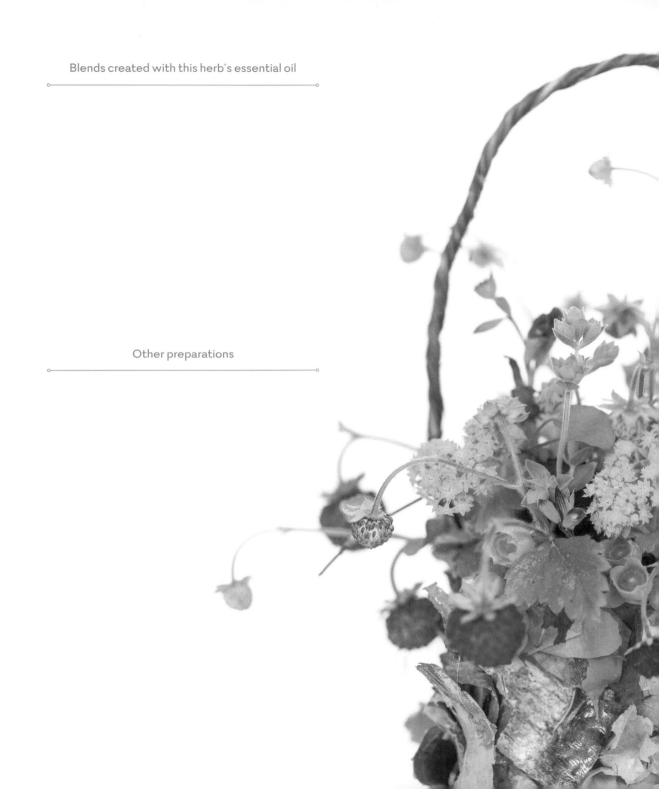

COMMON NAME
_____

BOTANICAL NAME   DATE

— ꙮ ꙮ ꙮ ꙮ —

Parts used

_____
_____
_____
_____

Notes on the plant or harvest

_____
_____
_____
_____

Recipes or medicines created

_____
_____
_____
_____
_____
_____
_____
_____
_____
_____

Blends created with this herb's essential oil

Other preparations

_____

COMMON NAME

_____   _____

BOTANICAL NAME   DATE

Parts used

_____

_____

_____

_____

Notes on the plant or harvest

_____

_____

_____

_____

Recipes or medicines created

_____

_____

_____

_____

_____

_____

_____

_____

_____

_____

Blends created with this herb's essential oil

Other preparations

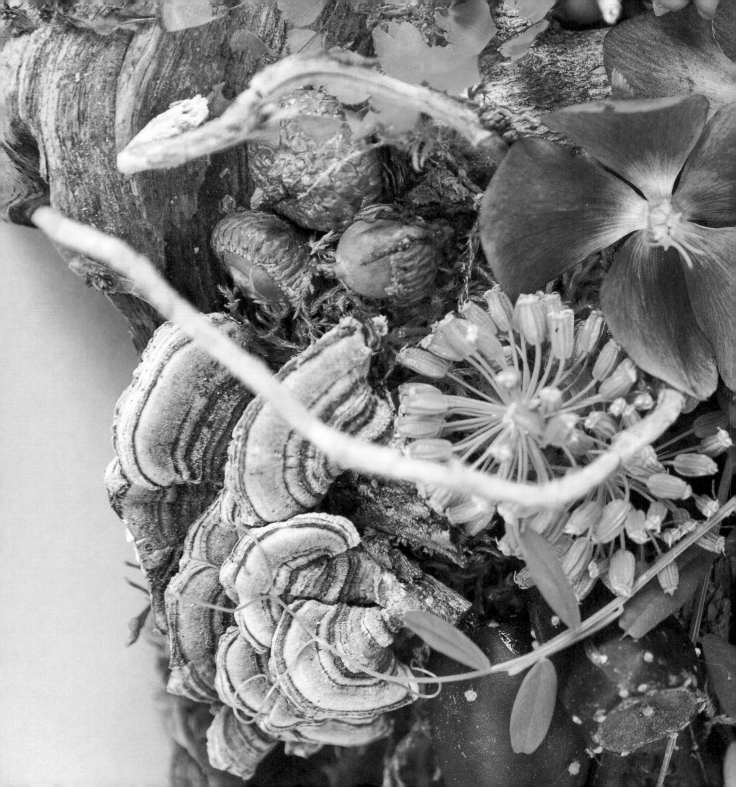

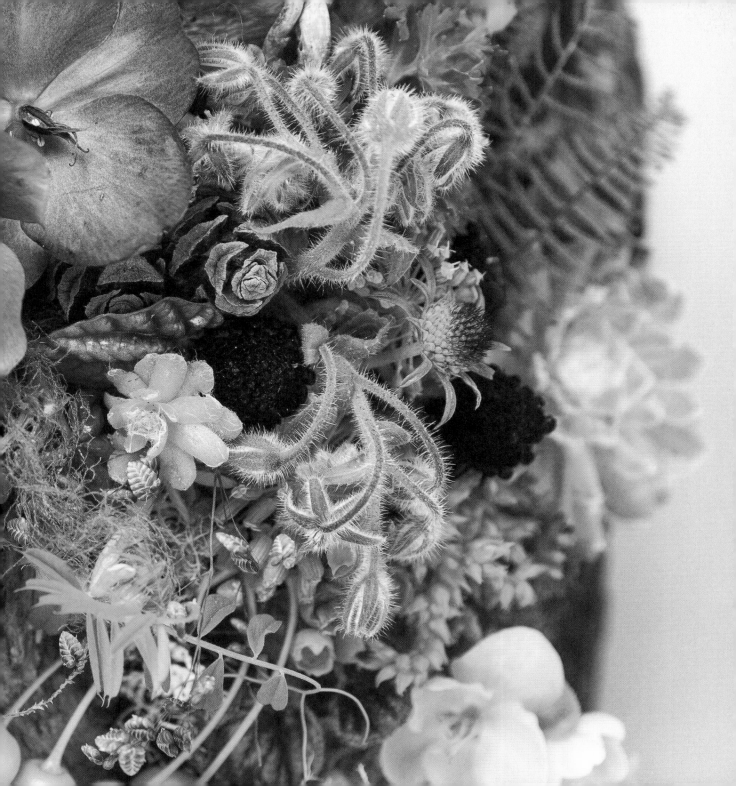

COMMON NAME

BOTANICAL NAME   DATE

⚬———— ✻⚬✻⚬✻ ✻⚬✻ ————⚬

Parts used   Notes on the plant or harvest

Recipes or medicines created

Blends created with this herb's essential oil

Other preparations

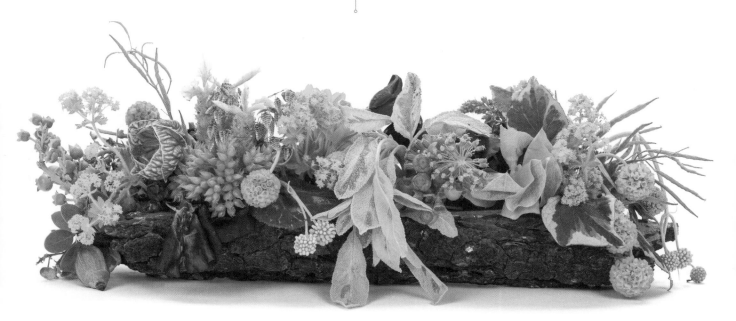

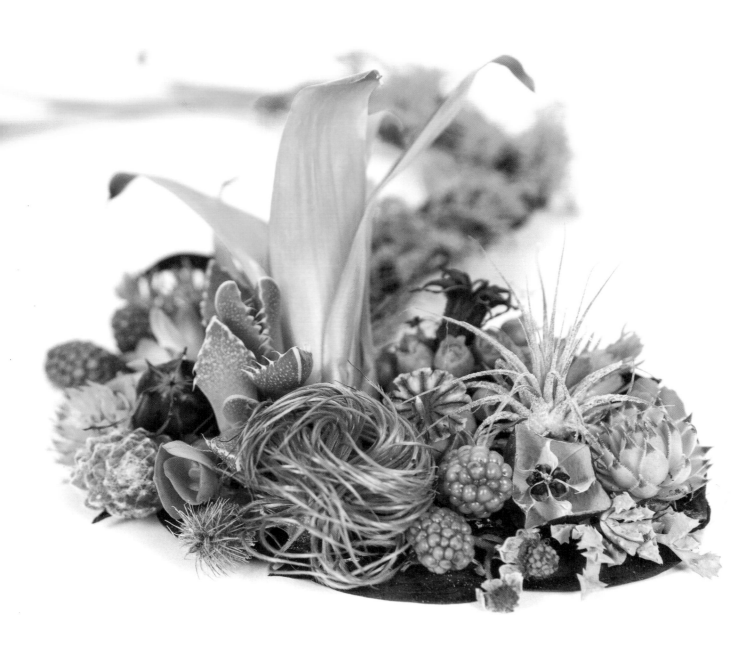

COMMON NAME

BOTANICAL NAME

DATE

— ⚘⚘⚘⚘ —

Parts used

Notes on the plant or harvest

Recipes or medicines created

Blends created with this herb's essential oil

Other preparations

Parts used

Notes on the plant or harvest

Recipes or medicines created

Blends created with this herb's essential oil

Other preparations

_____

COMMON NAME

_____

BOTANICAL NAME   DATE

— ⋅⊷⧬⊶⋅ —

Parts used   Notes on the plant or harvest

_____   _____
_____   _____
_____   _____
_____

                                        Recipes or medicines created

                                        _____
                                        _____
                                        _____
                                        _____
                                        _____
                                        _____
                                        _____

                                        _____

                                        _____

34

Blends created with this herb's essential oil

Other preparations

COMMON NAME

BOTANICAL NAME

DATE

Parts used

Notes on the plant or harvest

Recipes or medicines created

Blends created with this herb's essential oil

Other preparations

_____

COMMON NAME

_____   _____

BOTANICAL NAME   DATE

—— ⁍⁌⁍⁌⁍⁌ ——

Parts used

_____

_____

_____

_____

Notes on the plant or harvest

_____

_____

_____

_____

Recipes or medicines created

_____

_____

_____

_____

_____

_____

_____

_____

_____

_____

Blends created with this herb's essential oil

Other preparations

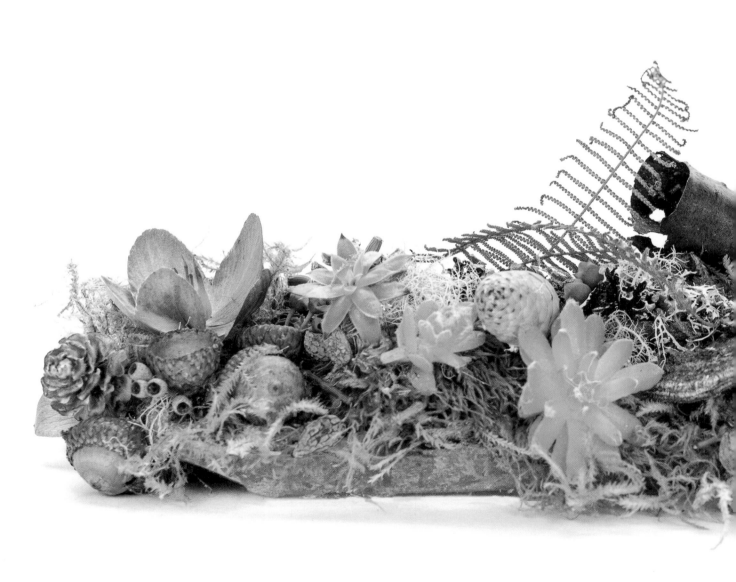

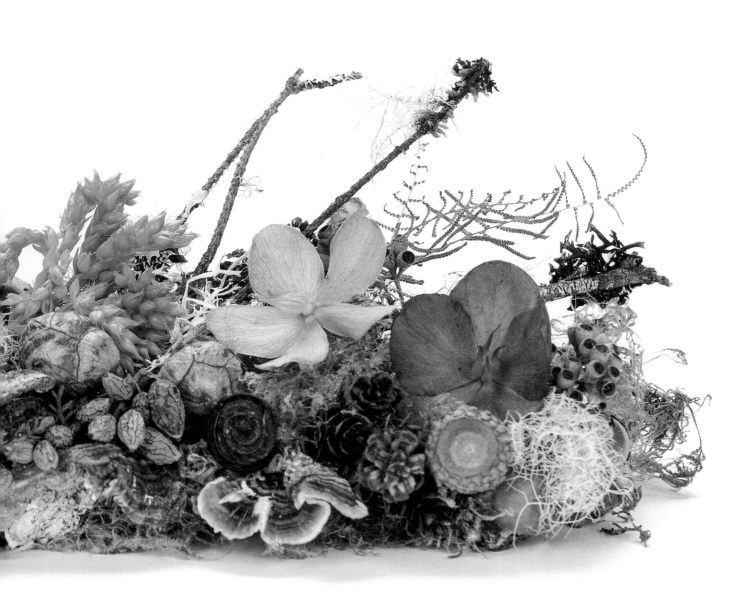

COMMON NAME

BOTANICAL NAME

DATE

Parts used

Notes on the plant or harvest

Recipes or medicines created

Blends created with this herb's essential oil

Other preparations

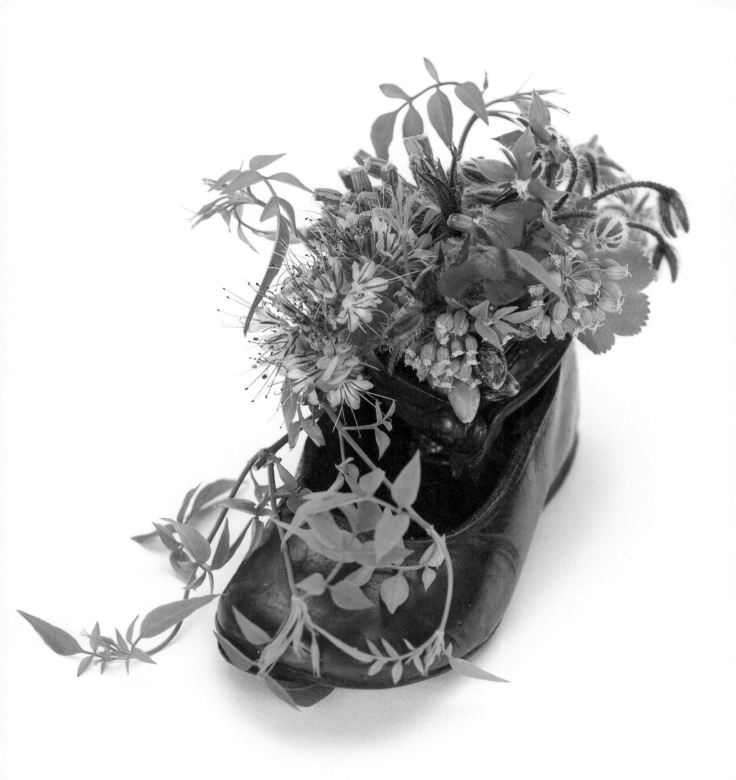

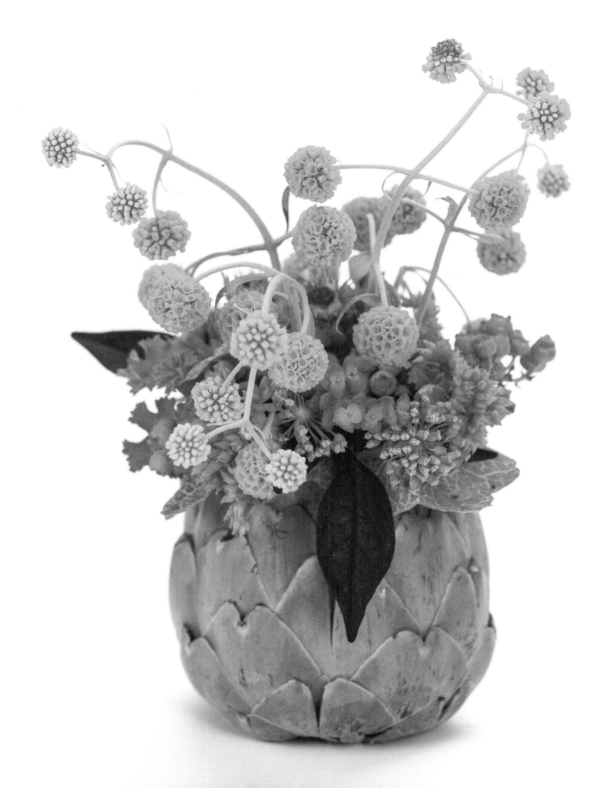

COMMON NAME

BOTANICAL NAME   DATE

— ❧—⚘⚘⚘⚘⚘—❧ —

Parts used   Notes on the plant or harvest

_____   _____
_____   _____
_____   _____
_____   _____

Recipes or medicines created   Blends created with this herb's essential oil

_____
_____
_____
_____
_____   Other preparations
_____
_____
_____
_____
_____

_____

COMMON NAME

_____   _____

BOTANICAL NAME   DATE

Parts used   Notes on the plant or harvest

_____   _____
_____   _____
_____   _____
_____   _____

Recipes or medicines created

_____
_____
_____
_____
_____
_____
_____
_____
_____
_____
_____

Blends created with this herb's essential oil

Other preparations

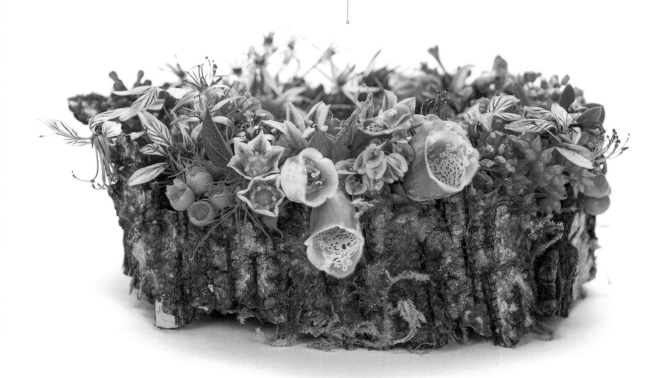

COMMON NAME

BOTANICAL NAME   DATE

❧ ⟶ ⟵ ❧

Parts used   Notes on the plant or harvest

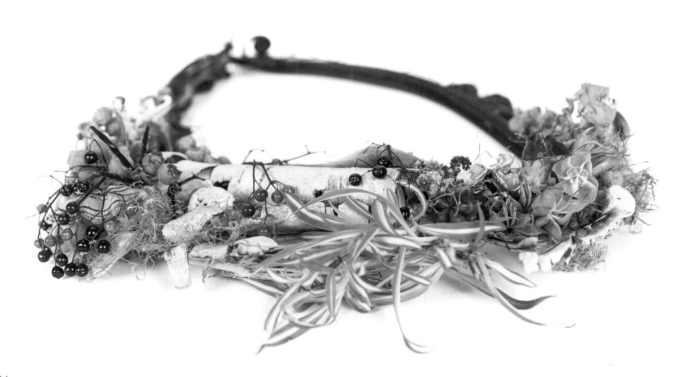

Recipes or medicines created

_____
_____
_____
_____
_____
_____
_____
_____
_____
_____

Blends created with this herb's essential oil

Other preparations

_____

COMMON NAME

_____   _____

BOTANICAL NAME   DATE

— ❧ ❧❧❧❧ ❧❧ ❧ —

Parts used   Notes on the plant or harvest

_____   _____

_____   _____

_____   _____

_____   _____

Recipes or medicines created

_____

_____

_____

_____

_____

_____

_____

_____

_____

_____

_____

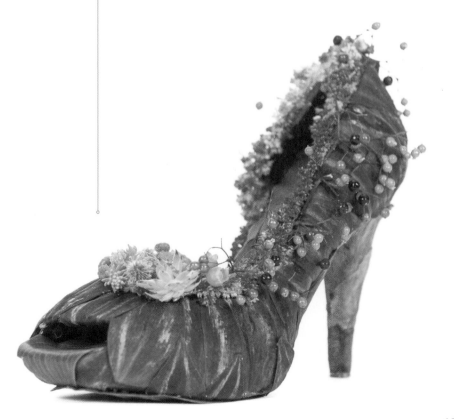

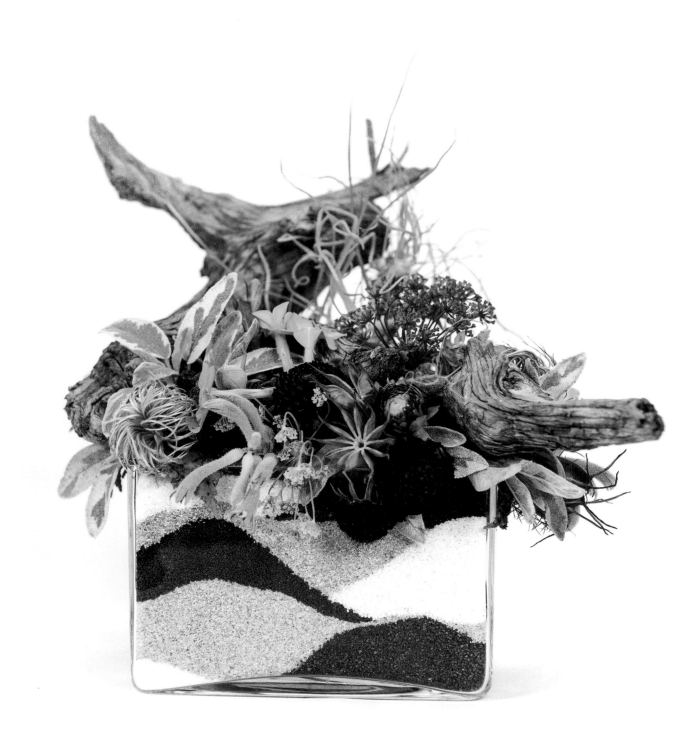

_____

COMMON NAME

_____   _____

BOTANICAL NAME   DATE

Parts used

_____
_____
_____
_____

Notes on the plant or harvest

_____
_____
_____
_____

Recipes or medicines created

_____
_____
_____
_____
_____
_____
_____
_____
_____
_____

Blends created with this herb's essential oil

Other preparations

COMMON NAME

BOTANICAL NAME

DATE

Parts used

Notes on the plant or harvest

Recipes or medicines created

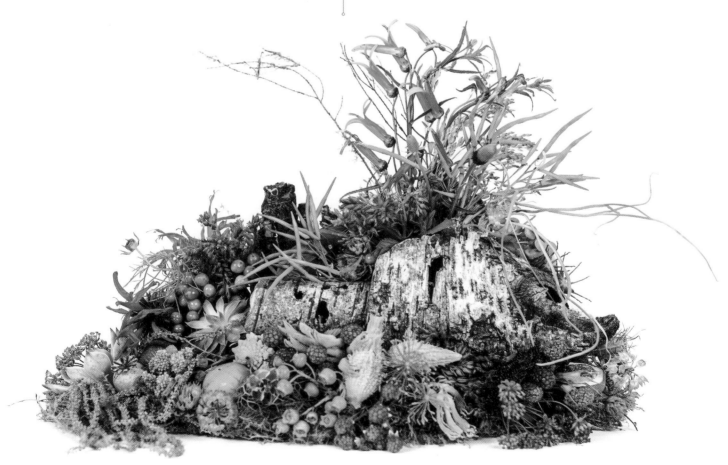

COMMON NAME

BOTANICAL NAME

DATE

Parts used

Notes on the plant or harvest

Recipes or medicines created

Blends created with this herb's essential oil

Other preparations

_____

COMMON NAME

_____

BOTANICAL NAME   DATE

Parts used

_____
_____
_____
_____

Notes on the plant or harvest

_____
_____
_____
_____

Recipes or medicines created

_____
_____
_____
_____
_____
_____
_____
_____
_____
_____

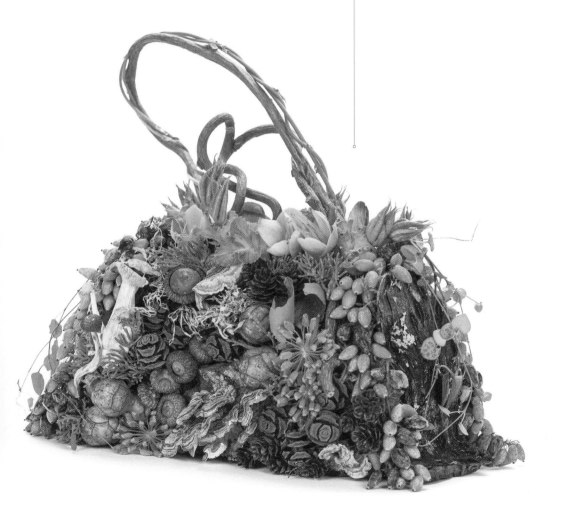

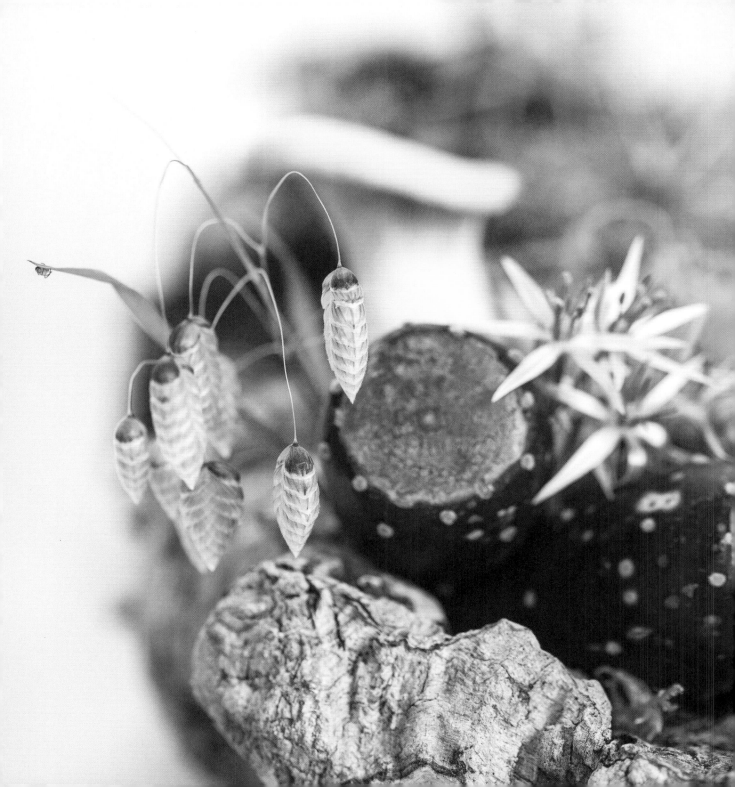

_____

COMMON NAME

_____   _____

BOTANICAL NAME   DATE

❧ ——— ⁕⁂⁕⁂⁕ ——— ❧

Parts used

_____
_____
_____
_____

Notes on the plant or harvest

_____
_____
_____
_____

Recipes or medicines created

_____
_____
_____
_____
_____
_____
_____
_____
_____
_____

Blends created with this herb's essential oil

Other preparations

COMMON NAME

BOTANICAL NAME

DATE

Parts used

Notes on the plant or harvest

Recipes or medicines created

Blends created with this herb's essential oil

Other preparations

COMMON NAME

BOTANICAL NAME

DATE

Parts used

Notes on the plant or harvest

Recipes or medicines created

Blends created with this herb's essential oil   Other preparations

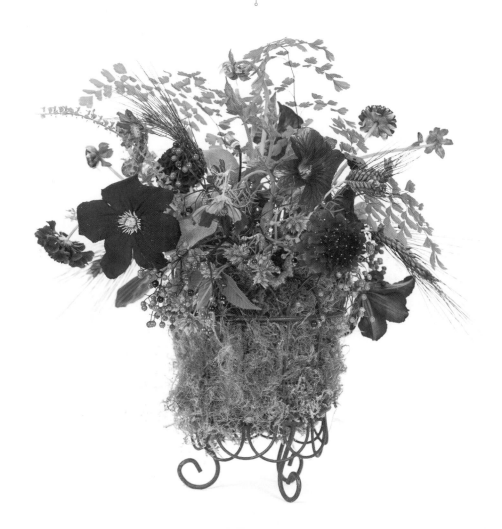

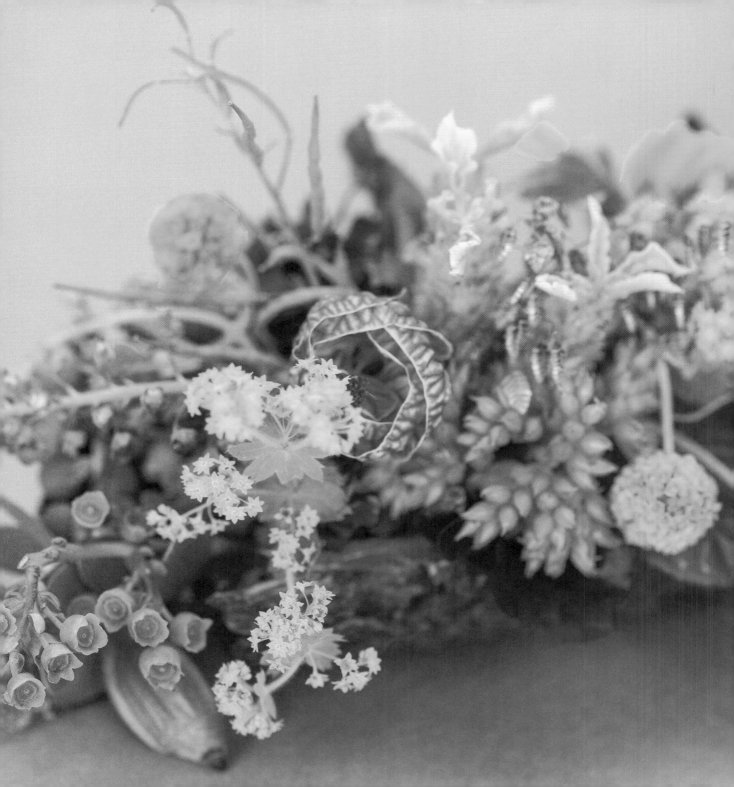

_____

COMMON NAME

_____   _____

BOTANICAL NAME   DATE

Parts used

_____
_____
_____
_____

Notes on the plant or harvest

_____
_____
_____
_____

Recipes or medicines created

_____
_____
_____
_____
_____
_____
_____
_____
_____
_____

Blends created with this herb's essential oil

Other preparations

_____

COMMON NAME

_____   _____

BOTANICAL NAME   DATE

Parts used

_____
_____
_____
_____

Notes on the plant or harvest

_____
_____
_____
_____

Recipes or medicines created

_____
_____
_____
_____
_____
_____
_____
_____
_____
_____

Blends created with this herb's essential oil

Other preparations

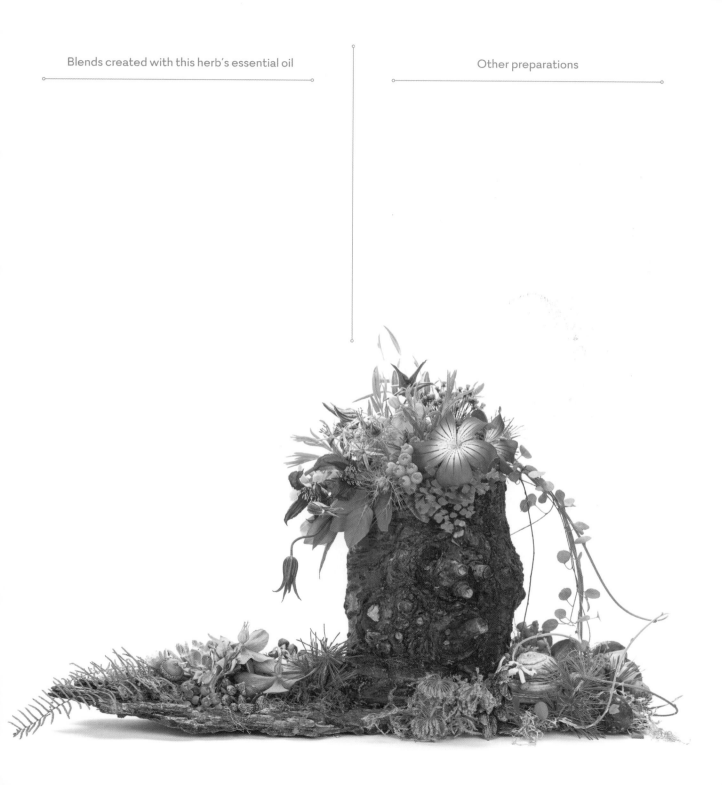

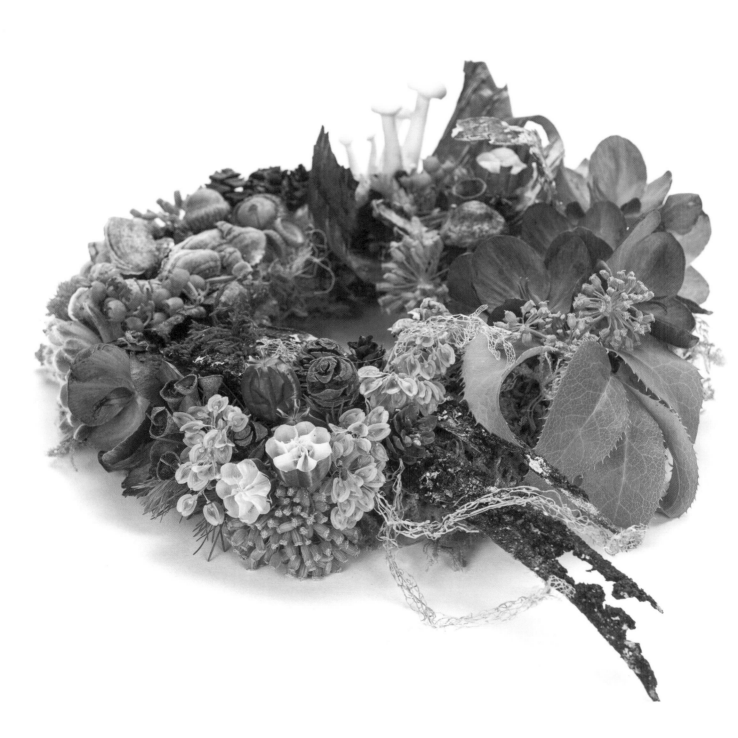

COMMON NAME

BOTANICAL NAME

DATE

Parts used

Notes on the plant or harvest

Recipes or medicines created

Blends created with this herb's essential oil

Other preparations

COMMON NAME

BOTANICAL NAME

DATE

Parts used

Notes on the plant or harvest

Recipes or medicines created

Blends created with this herb's essential oil

Other preparations

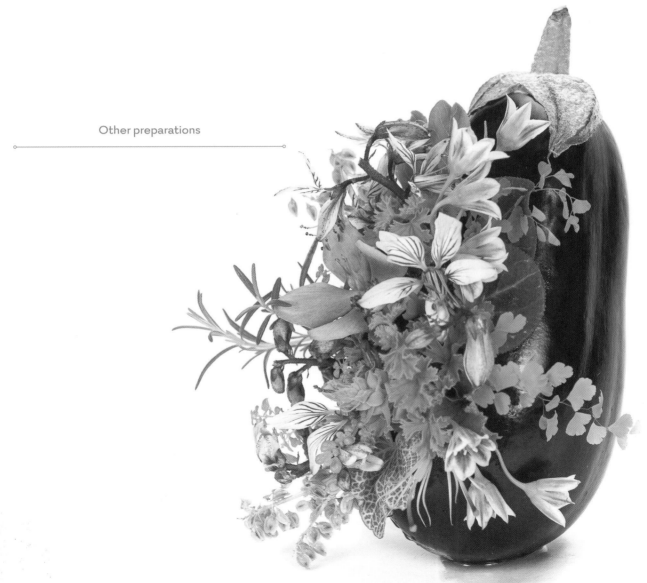

COMMON NAME

BOTANICAL NAME

DATE

Parts used

Notes on the plant or harvest

Recipes or medicines created

Blends created with this herb's essential oil

Other preparations

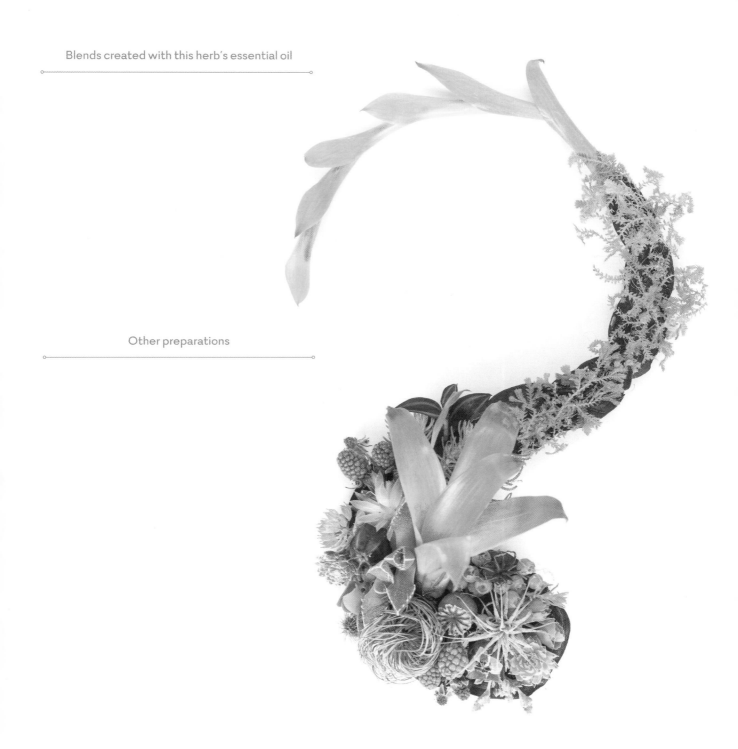

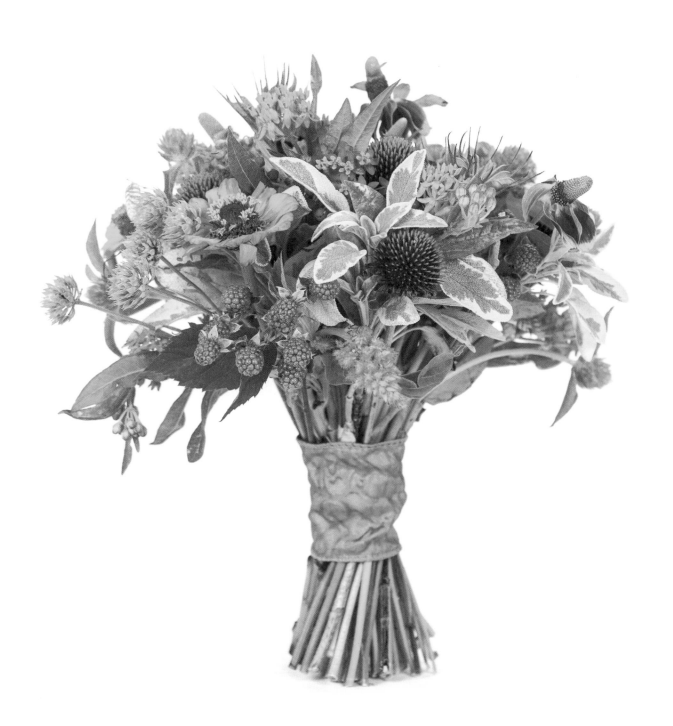

_____

COMMON NAME

_____   _____

BOTANICAL NAME   DATE

Parts used

_____
_____
_____
_____

Notes on the plant or harvest

_____
_____
_____
_____

Recipes or medicines created

_____
_____
_____
_____
_____
_____
_____
_____
_____
_____

Blends created with this herb's essential oil

Other preparations

_____

COMMON NAME

_____   _____

BOTANICAL NAME   DATE

Parts used

_____
_____
_____
_____

Notes on the plant or harvest

_____
_____
_____
_____

Recipes or medicines created

_____
_____
_____
_____
_____
_____
_____
_____
_____
_____

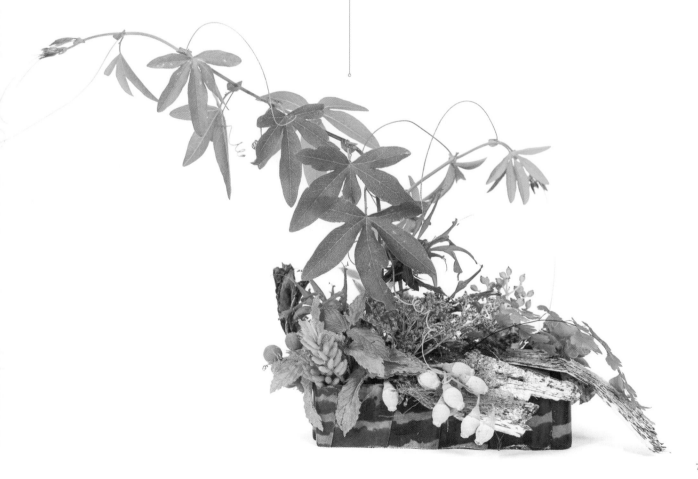

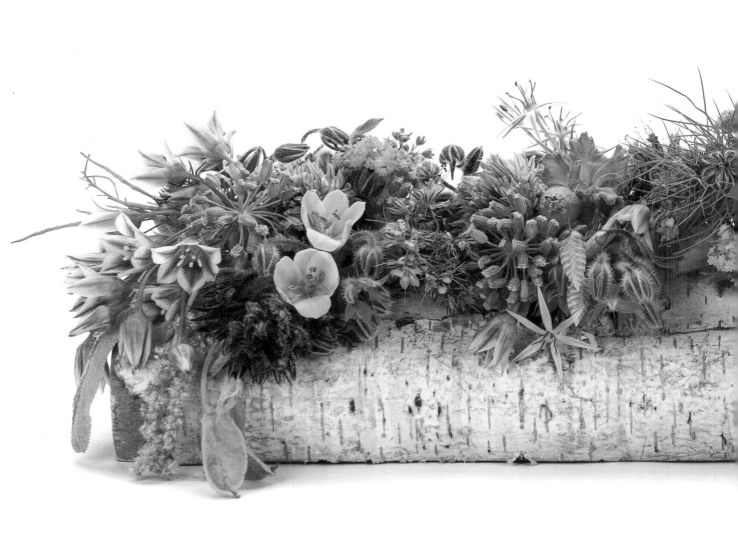

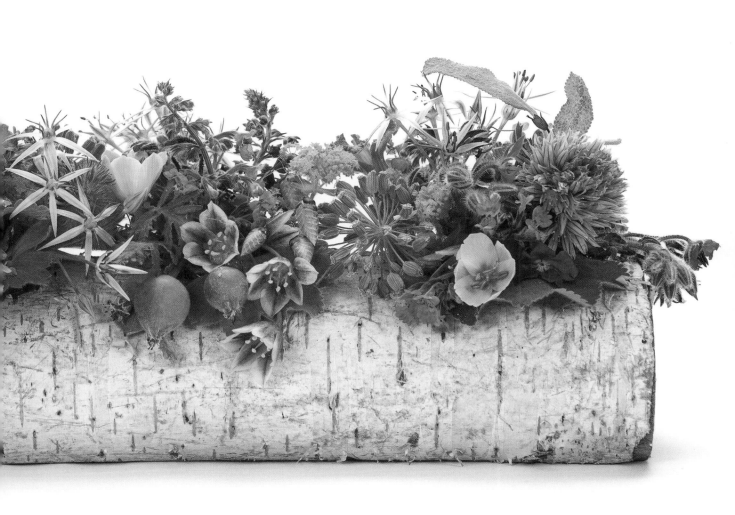

_____

COMMON NAME

_____   _____

BOTANICAL NAME   DATE

Parts used   Notes on the plant or harvest

_____   _____
_____   _____
_____   _____
_____   _____

Recipes or medicines created   Blends created with this herb's essential oil

_____
_____
_____
_____
_____
_____   Other preparations
_____
_____
_____
_____
_____

COMMON NAME

BOTANICAL NAME

DATE

Parts used

Notes on the plant or harvest

Recipes or medicines created

Blends created with this herb's essential oil

Other preparations

_____

COMMON NAME

_____

BOTANICAL NAME   DATE

Parts used

_____
_____
_____
_____

Notes on the plant or harvest

_____
_____
_____
_____

Recipes or medicines created

_____
_____
_____
_____
_____
_____
_____
_____
_____
_____

Blends created with this herb's essential oil

Other preparations

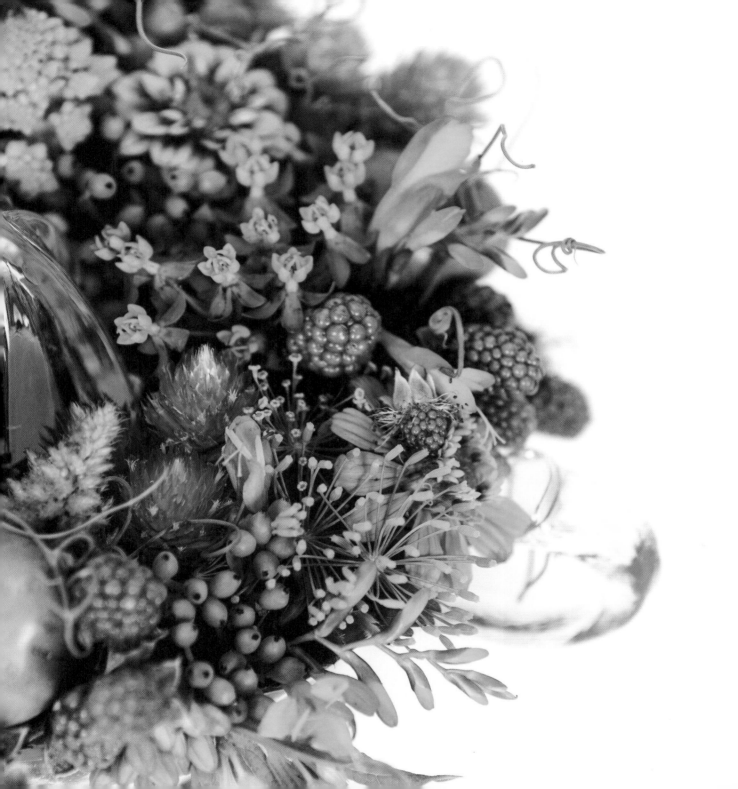

COMMON NAME

BOTANICAL NAME

DATE

Parts used

Notes on the plant or harvest

Recipes or medicines created

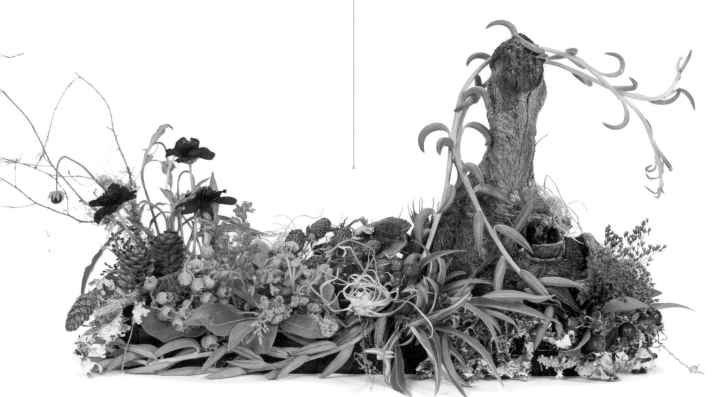

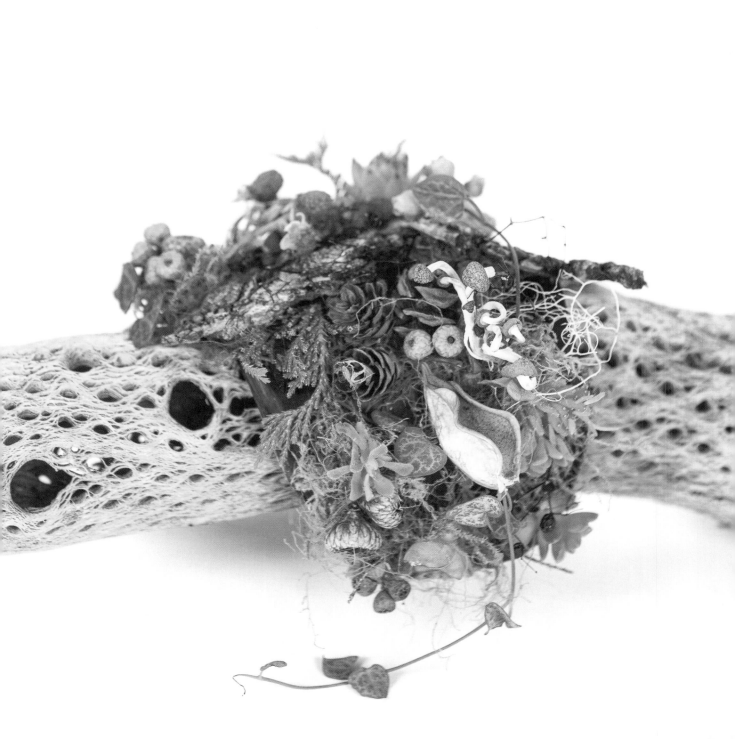

_____

COMMON NAME

_____   _____

BOTANICAL NAME   DATE

Parts used

_____
_____
_____
_____

Notes on the plant or harvest

_____
_____
_____
_____

Recipes or medicines created

_____
_____
_____
_____
_____
_____
_____
_____
_____
_____

Blends created with this herb's essential oil

Other preparations

COMMON NAME

BOTANICAL NAME

DATE

Parts used

Notes on the plant or harvest

Recipes or medicines created

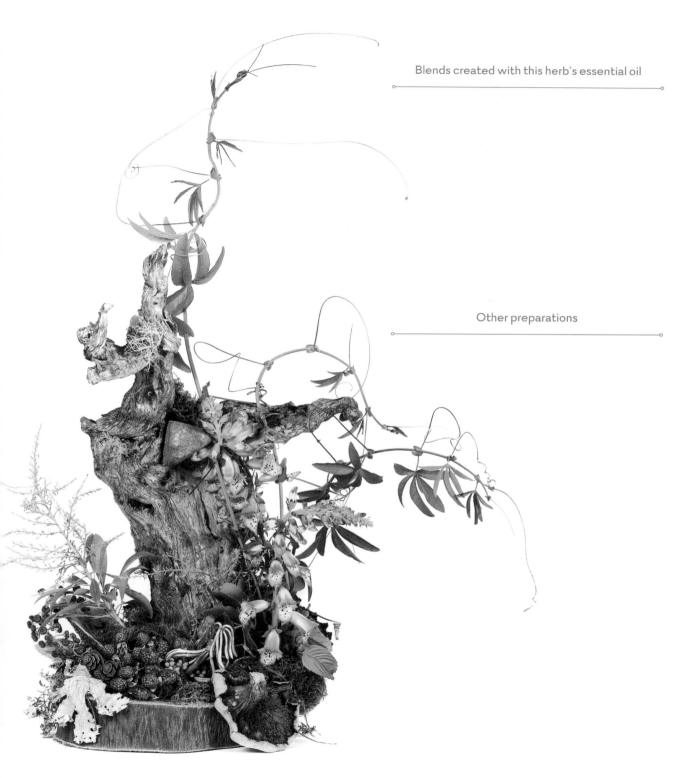

Blends created with this herb's essential oil

Other preparations

COMMON NAME

BOTANICAL NAME

DATE

Parts used

Notes on the plant or harvest

Recipes or medicines created

Blends created with this herb's essential oil

Other preparations

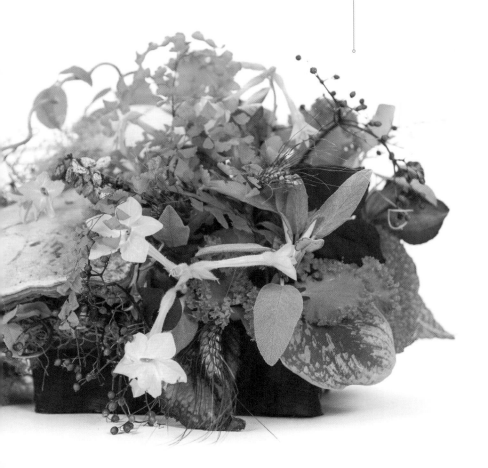

COMMON NAME

BOTANICAL NAME

DATE

Parts used

Notes on the plant or harvest

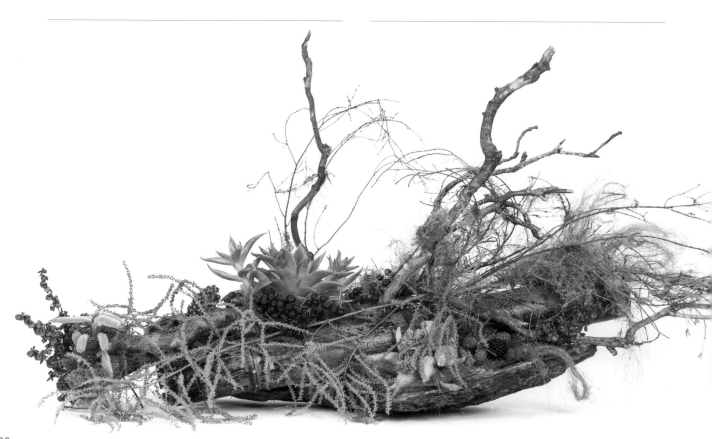

Recipes or medicines created

Blends created with this herb's essential oil

Other preparations

COMMON NAME

BOTANICAL NAME

DATE

Parts used

Notes on the plant or harvest

Recipes or medicines created

Blends created with this herb's essential oil

Other preparations

_____

COMMON NAME

_____

BOTANICAL NAME   DATE

— ❧ ⬥❧⬥❧⬥ ❧ —

Parts used   Notes on the plant or harvest

_____   _____
_____   _____
_____   _____
_____   _____

Recipes or medicines created   Blends created with this herb's essential oil

_____
_____
_____
_____
_____   Other preparations
_____
_____
_____
_____

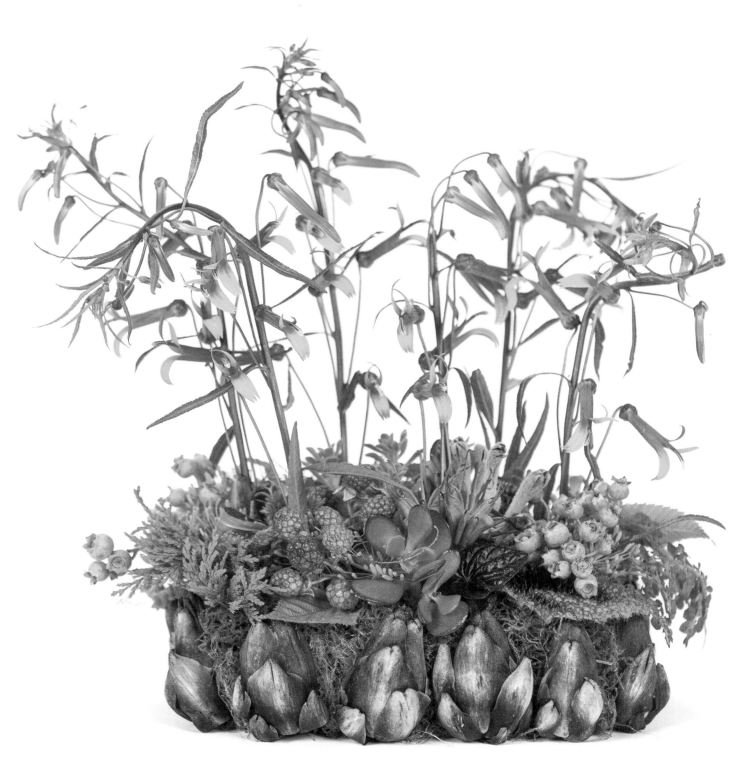

_____

COMMON NAME

_____   _____

BOTANICAL NAME   DATE

———— ⚜ ————

Parts used

_____

_____

_____

_____

Notes on the plant or harvest

_____

_____

_____

_____

Recipes or medicines created

_____

_____

_____

_____

_____

_____

_____

_____

_____

Blends created with this herb's essential oil

Other preparations

COMMON NAME

BOTANICAL NAME

DATE

Parts used

Notes on the plant or harvest

Recipes or medicines created

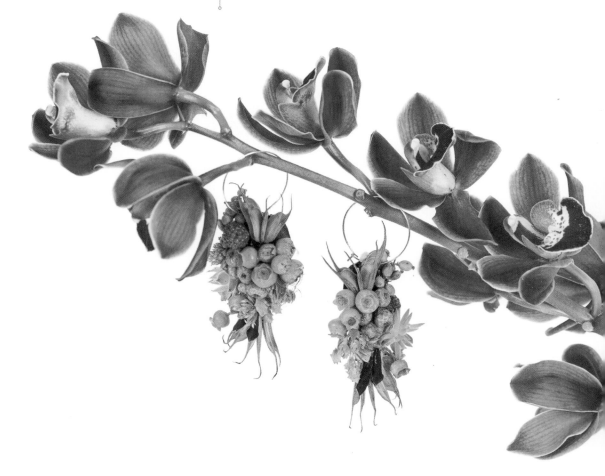

Blends created with this herb's essential oil

Other preparations

99

COMMON NAME

BOTANICAL NAME

DATE

⸙

Parts used

Notes on the plant or harvest

Recipes or medicines created

Blends created with this herb's essential oil

Other preparations

COMMON NAME

BOTANICAL NAME   DATE

—⁓ ⋅⊰⊹⊱⋅ ⊰⊹⊱⋅⊰⊹⊱ ⁓—

Parts used   Notes on the plant or harvest

Recipes or medicines created   Blends created with this herb's essential oil

Other preparations

COMMON NAME

BOTANICAL NAME

DATE

Parts used

Notes on the plant or harvest

Recipes or medicines created

Blends created with this herb's essential oil

Other preparations

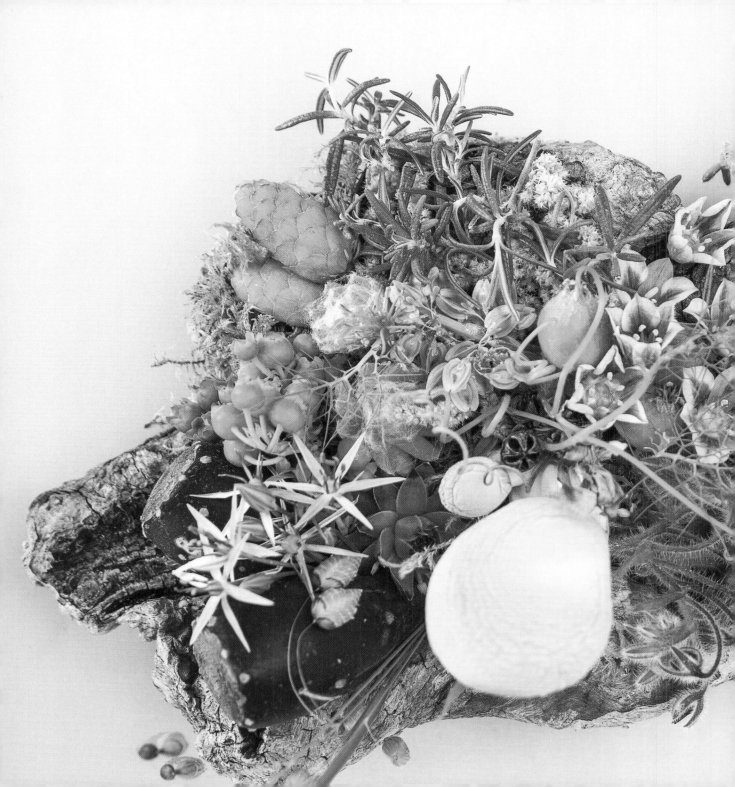

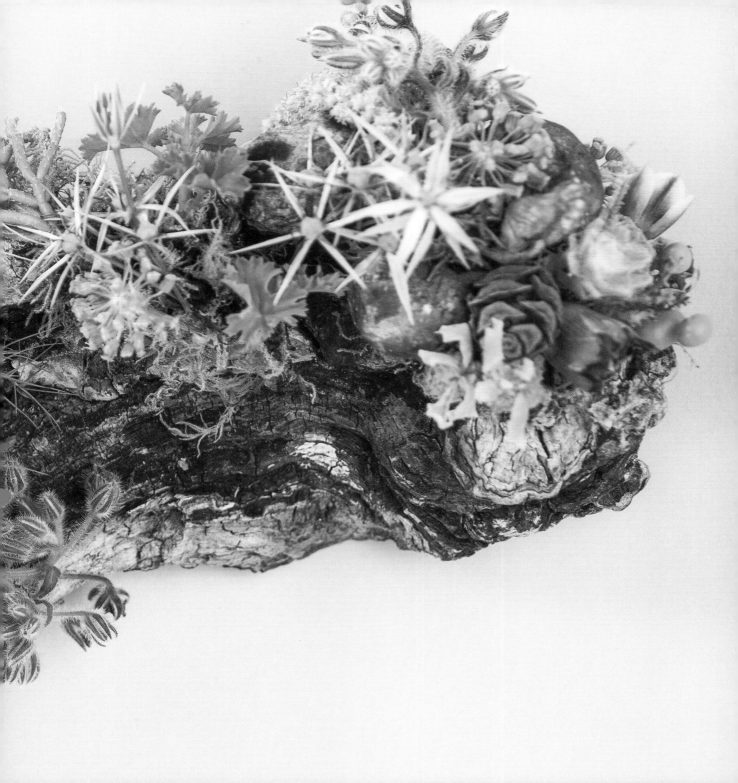

COMMON NAME

BOTANICAL NAME

DATE

Parts used

Notes on the plant or harvest

Recipes or medicines created

Blends created with this herb's essential oil

Other preparations

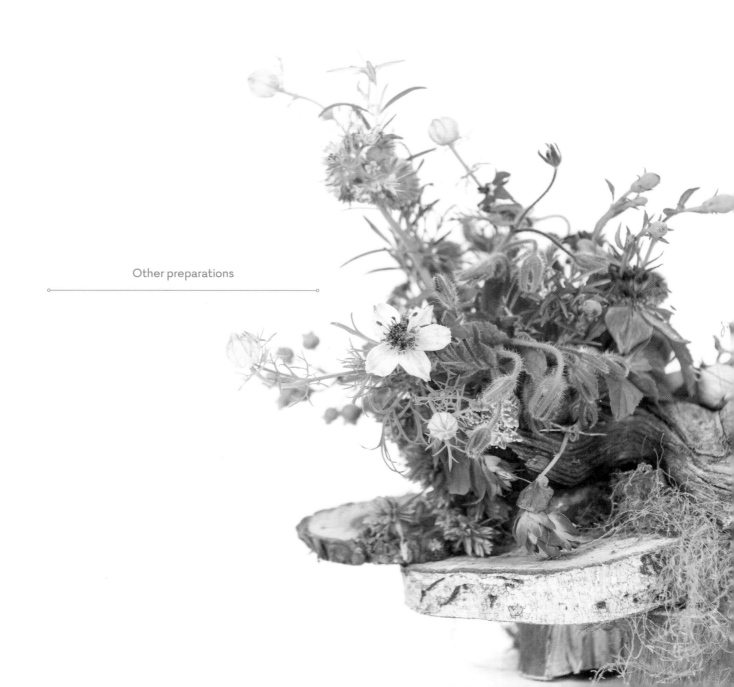

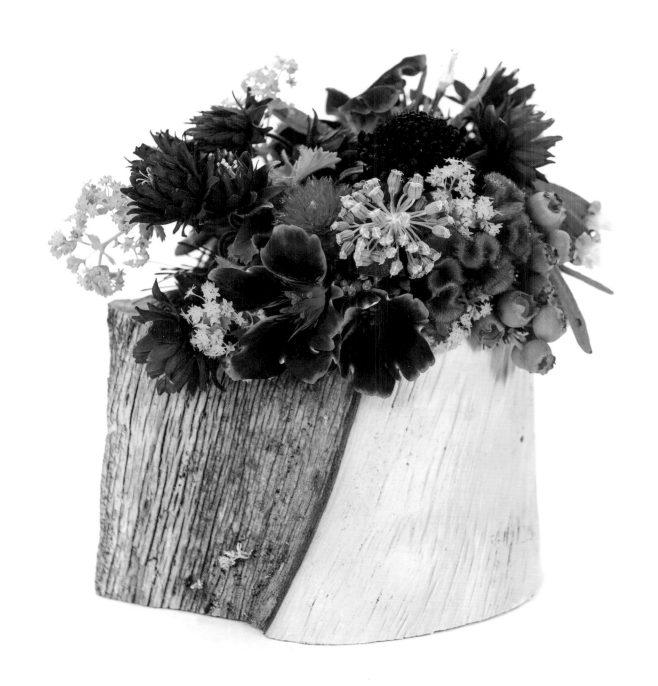

_____

COMMON NAME

_____   _____

BOTANICAL NAME   DATE

❧ ⸻ ❦❧❦ ⸻ ❧

Parts used

_____
_____
_____
_____

Notes on the plant or harvest

_____
_____
_____
_____

Recipes or medicines created

_____
_____
_____
_____
_____
_____
_____
_____
_____
_____

Blends created with this herb's essential oil

Other preparations

COMMON NAME

BOTANICAL NAME

DATE

Parts used

Notes on the plant or harvest

Recipes or medicines created

Blends created with this herb's essential oil

Other preparations

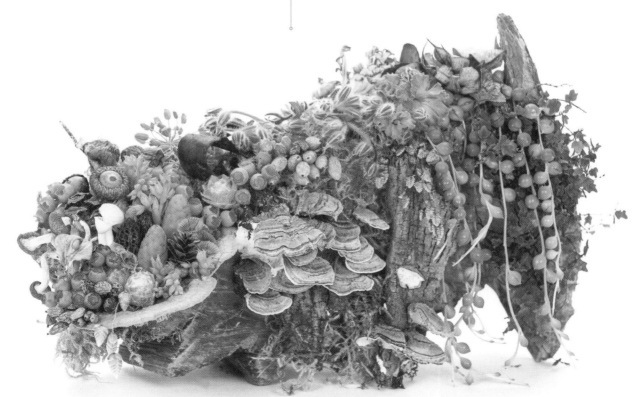

111

COMMON NAME

_____

BOTANICAL NAME   DATE

Parts used   Notes on the plant or harvest

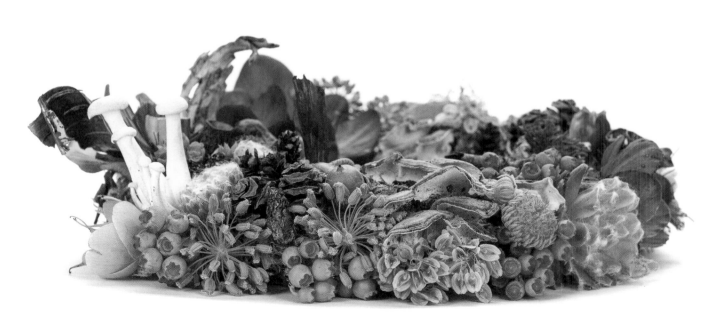

Recipes or medicines created

Blends created with this herb's essential oil

Other preparations

COMMON NAME

BOTANICAL NAME

DATE

Parts used

Notes on the plant or harvest

Recipes or medicines created

Blends created with this herb's essential oil

Other preparations

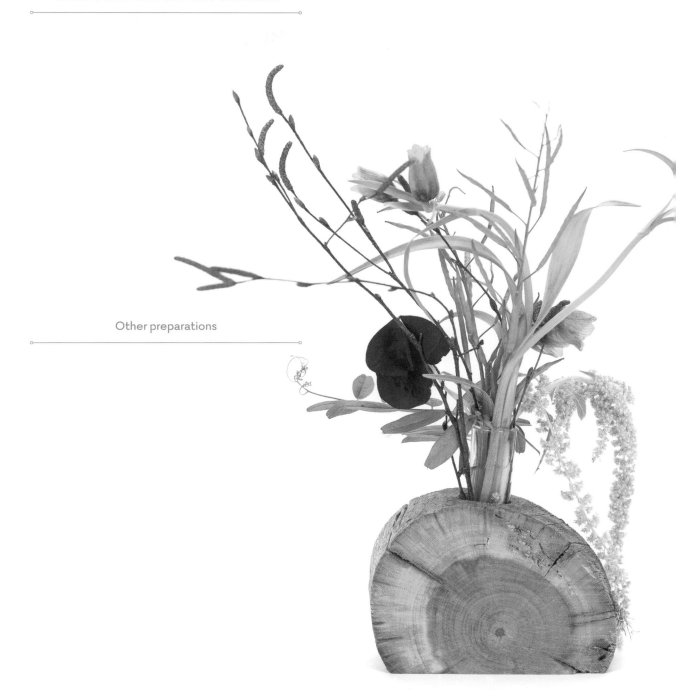

_____

COMMON NAME

_____

BOTANICAL NAME   DATE

Parts used

_____

_____

_____

_____

Notes on the plant or harvest

_____

_____

_____

_____

Recipes or medicines created

_____

_____

_____

_____

_____

_____

_____

_____

_____

_____

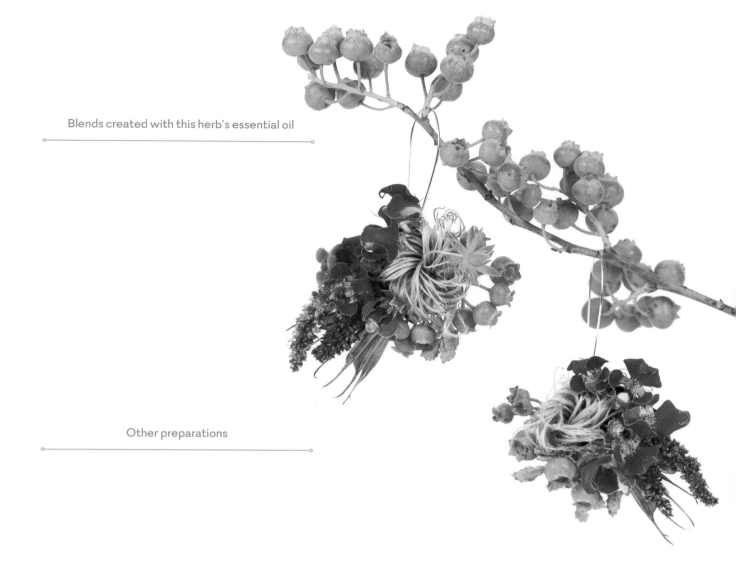

Blends created with this herb's essential oil

Other preparations

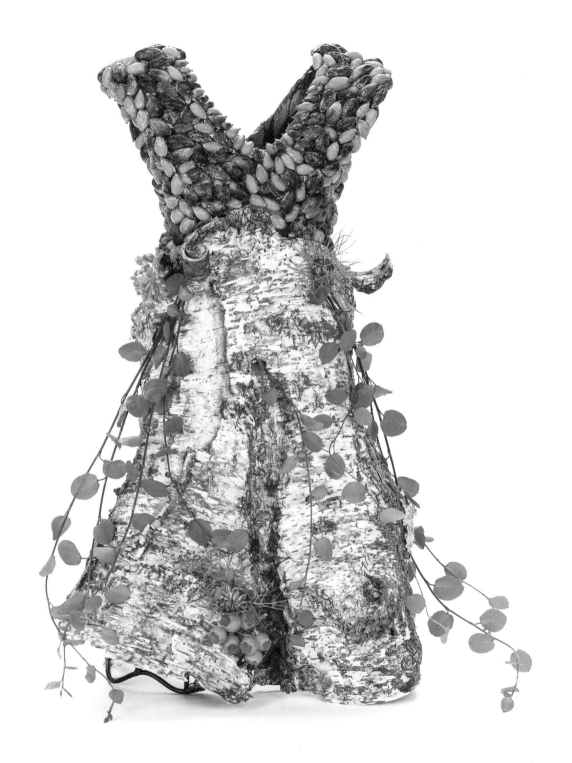

COMMON NAME

BOTANICAL NAME

DATE

Parts used

Notes on the plant or harvest

Recipes or medicines created

Blends created with this herb's essential oil

Other preparations

_____

COMMON NAME

_____   _____

BOTANICAL NAME   DATE

Parts used

_____
_____
_____
_____

Notes on the plant or harvest

_____
_____
_____
_____

Recipes or medicines created

_____
_____
_____
_____
_____
_____
_____
_____
_____
_____
_____

Blends created with this herb's essential oil

Other preparations

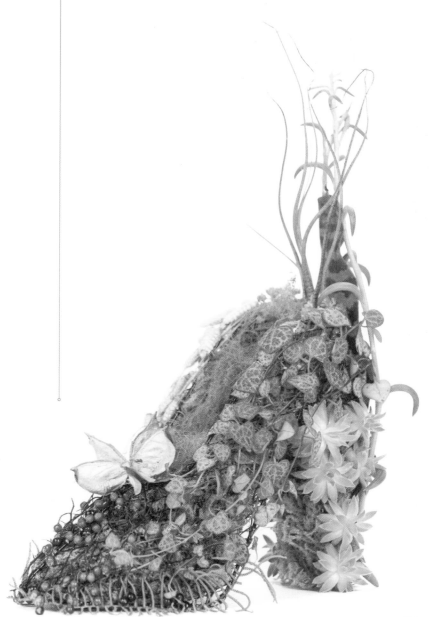

121

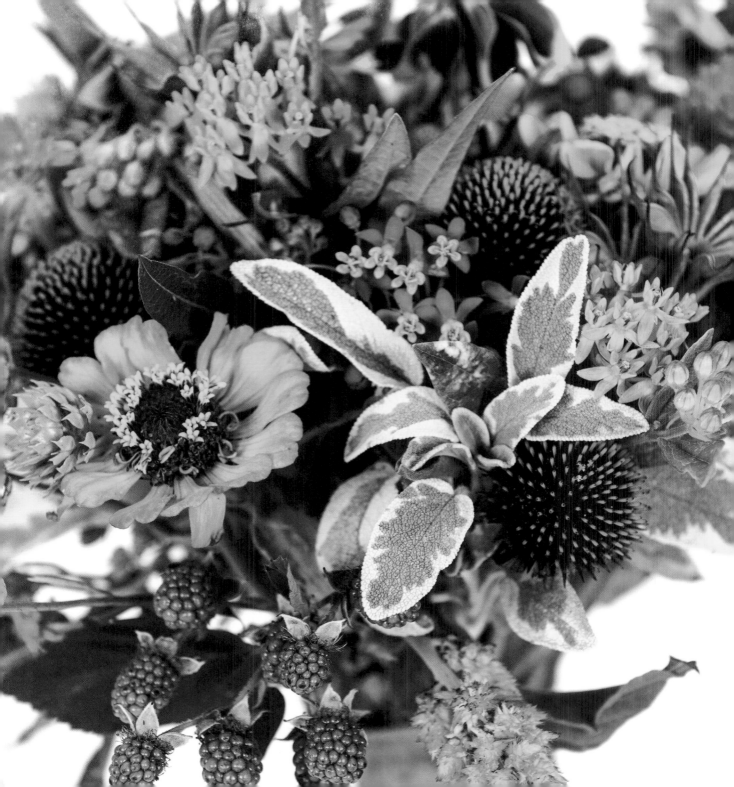

_____

COMMON NAME

_____   _____

BOTANICAL NAME   DATE

Parts used

_____

_____

_____

_____

Notes on the plant or harvest

_____

_____

_____

_____

Recipes or medicines created

_____

_____

_____

_____

_____

_____

_____

_____

_____

Blends created with this herb's essential oil

Other preparations

_____

COMMON NAME

_____

BOTANICAL NAME   DATE

— ❧ ❧ ❧ ❧ —

Parts used   Notes on the plant or harvest

_____   _____
_____   _____
_____   _____
_____   _____

Recipes or medicines created

_____
_____
_____
_____
_____
_____
_____
_____
_____
_____
_____

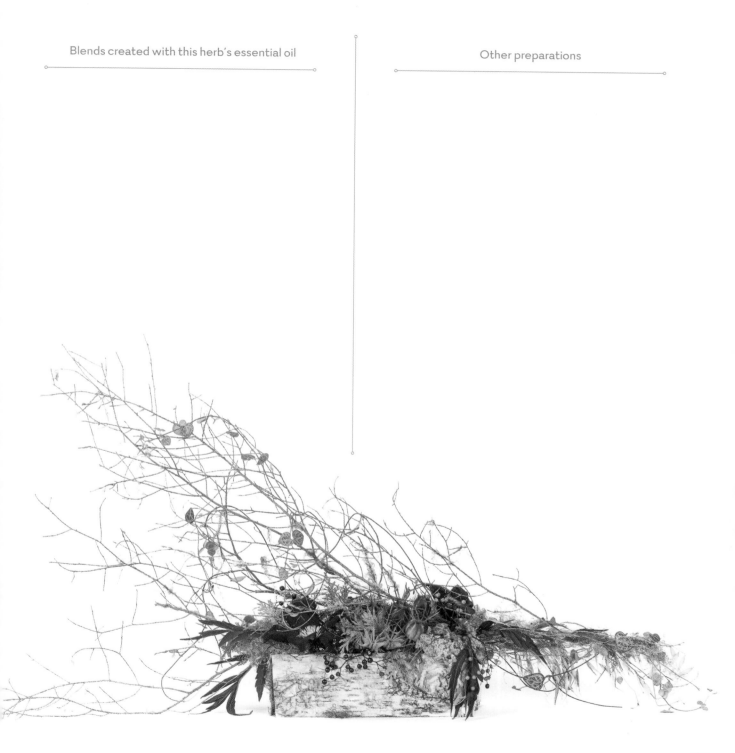

COMMON NAME

BOTANICAL NAME   DATE

❦ ⸝⸜⸌⸍⸝⸜ ❦

Parts used   Notes on the plant or harvest

Recipes or medicines created

Blends created with this herb's essential oil

Other preparations

COMMON NAME

BOTANICAL NAME

DATE

Parts used

Notes on the plant or harvest

Recipes or medicines created

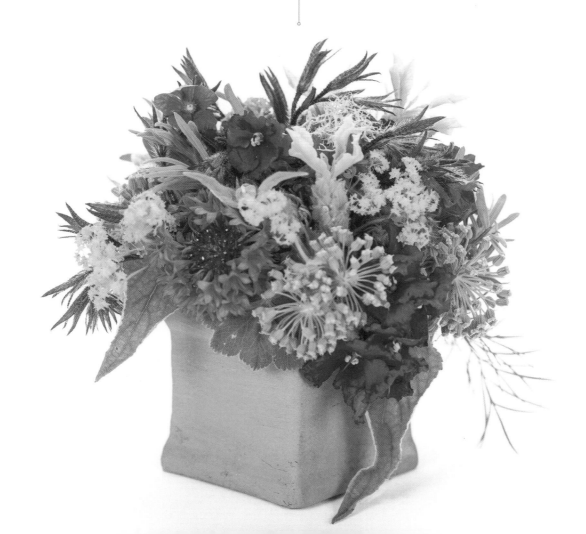

COMMON NAME

BOTANICAL NAME

DATE

Parts used

Notes on the plant or harvest

Recipes or medicines created

Blends created with this herb's essential oil

Other preparations

COMMON NAME

BOTANICAL NAME

DATE

Parts used

Notes on the plant or harvest

Recipes or medicines created

Blends created with this herb's essential oil

Other preparations

COMMON NAME

BOTANICAL NAME

DATE

Parts used

Notes on the plant or harvest

Recipes or medicines created

Blends created with this herb's essential oil

Other preparations

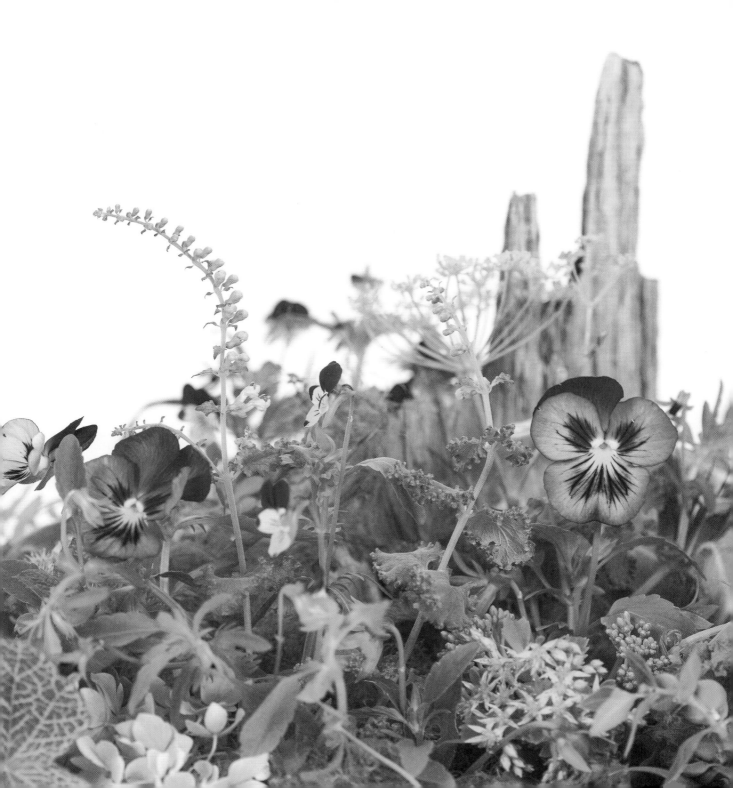

COMMON NAME

BOTANICAL NAME

DATE

Parts used

Notes on the plant or harvest

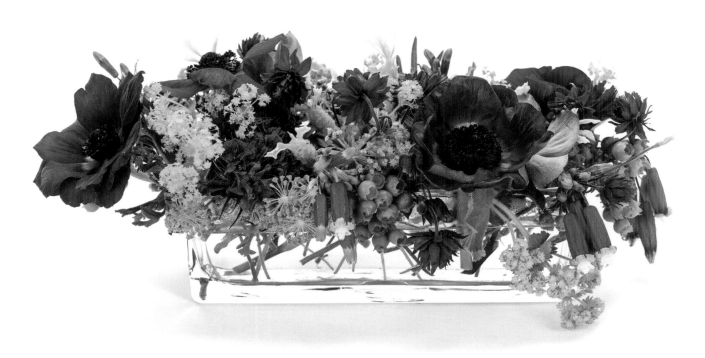

Recipes or medicines created

Blends created with this herb's essential oil

Other preparations

COMMON NAME

BOTANICAL NAME   DATE

Parts used   Notes on the plant or harvest

Recipes or medicines created   Blends created with this herb's essential oil

                                                  Other preparations

136

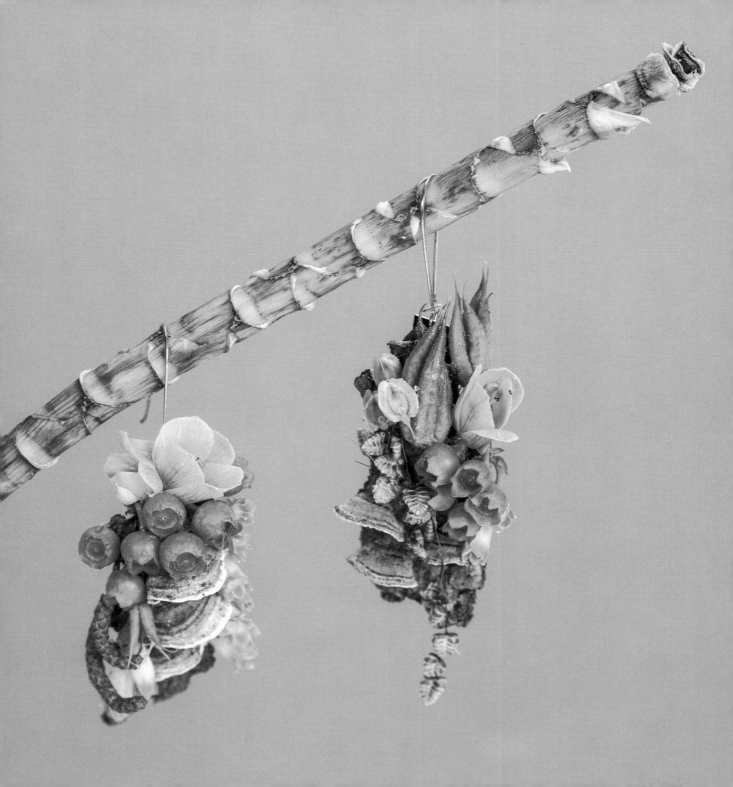

COMMON NAME

BOTANICAL NAME

DATE

⚬—⚭⚬⚭⚬⚭—⚬

Parts used

Notes on the plant or harvest

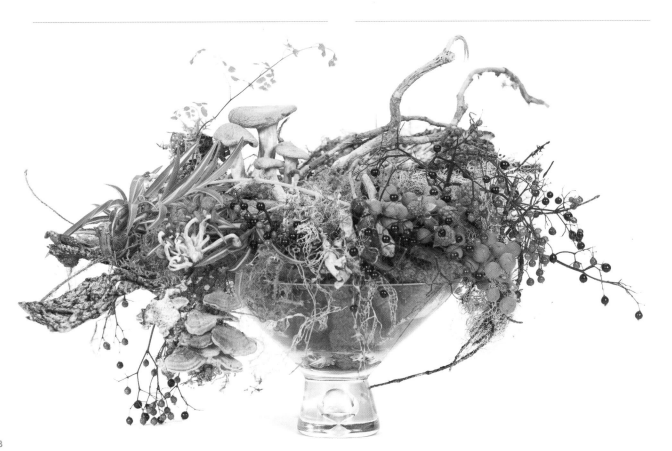

Recipes or medicines created

Blends created with this herb's essential oil

Other preparations

COMMON NAME

BOTANICAL NAME

DATE

Parts used

Notes on the plant or harvest

Recipes or medicines created

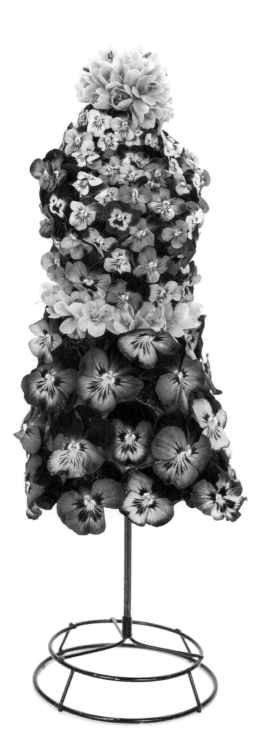

Blends created with this herb's essential oil

Other preparations

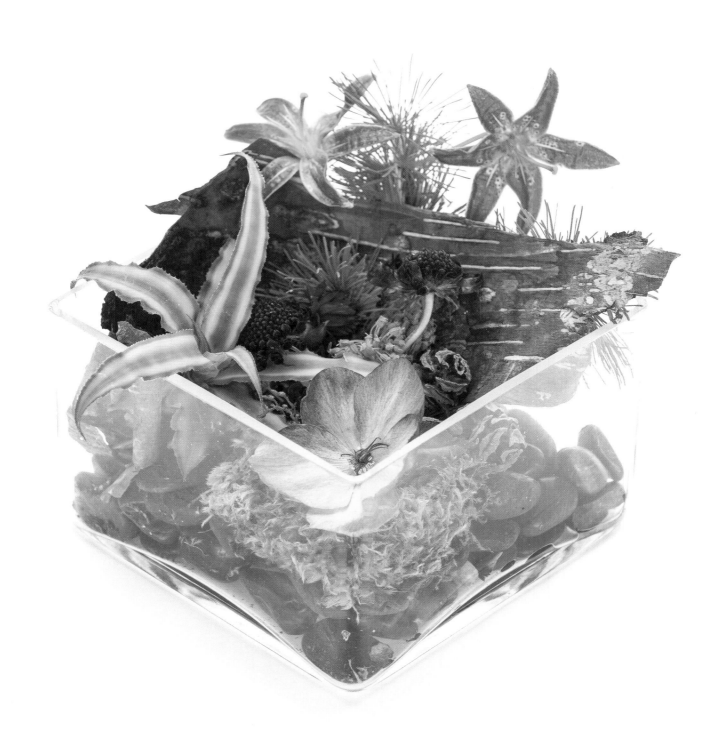

COMMON NAME

BOTANICAL NAME

DATE

Parts used

Notes on the plant or harvest

Recipes or medicines created

Blends created with this herb's essential oil

Other preparations

_____

COMMON NAME

_____   _____

BOTANICAL NAME   DATE

Parts used

_____
_____
_____
_____

Notes on the plant or harvest

_____
_____
_____
_____

Recipes or medicines created

_____
_____
_____
_____
_____
_____
_____
_____
_____
_____

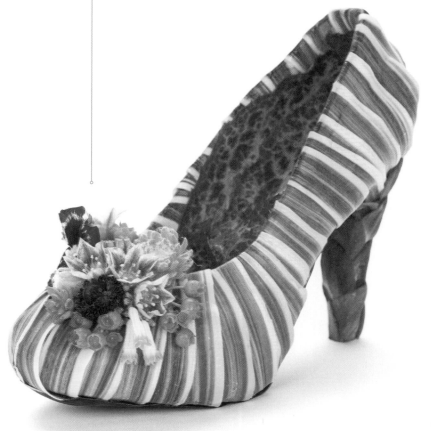

COMMON NAME

BOTANICAL NAME   DATE

❧ ⁂ ❧

Parts used   Notes on the plant or harvest

_____   _____
_____   _____
_____   _____
_____   _____

Recipes or medicines created

_____
_____
_____
_____
_____
_____
_____
_____
_____
_____
_____

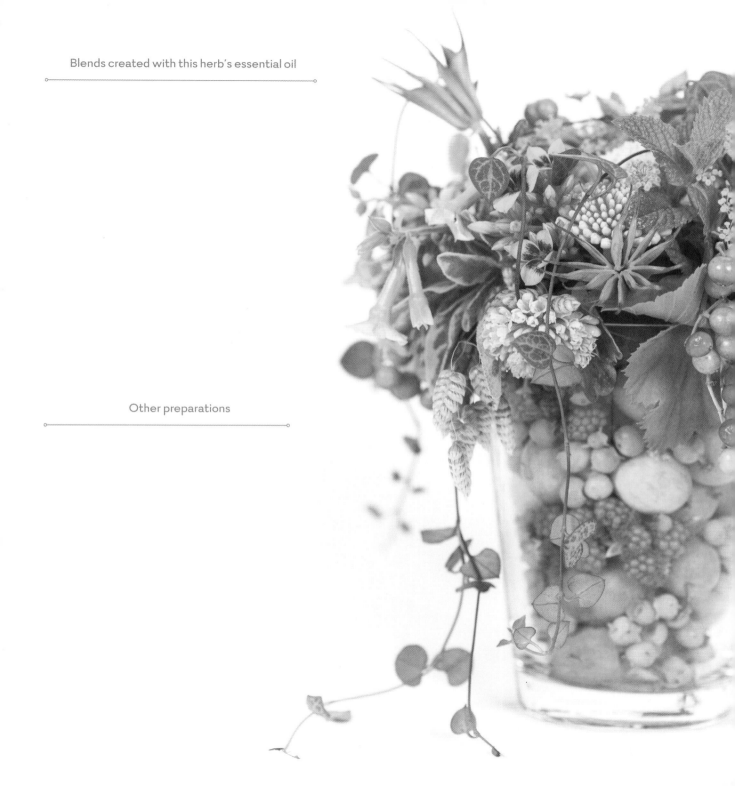

Blends created with this herb's essential oil

Other preparations

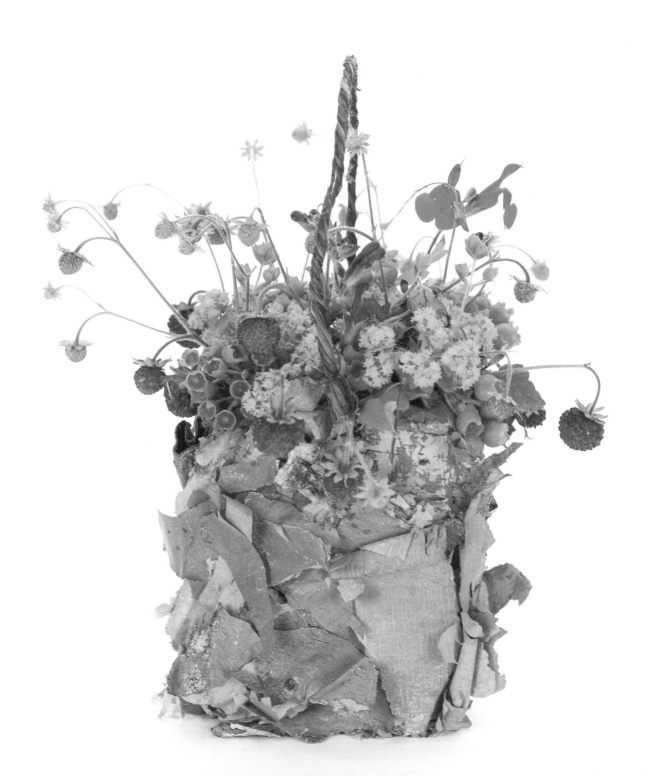

_____

COMMON NAME

_____

BOTANICAL NAME   DATE

—— ·❧❦❧· ——

Parts used

_____
_____
_____
_____

Notes on the plant or harvest

_____
_____
_____
_____

Recipes or medicines created

_____
_____
_____
_____
_____
_____
_____
_____
_____

Blends created with this herb's essential oil

Other preparations

_____

COMMON NAME

_____

BOTANICAL NAME   DATE

Parts used   Notes on the plant or harvest

_____   _____
_____   _____
_____   _____
_____   _____

Recipes or medicines created

_____
_____
_____
_____
_____
_____
_____
_____
_____
_____

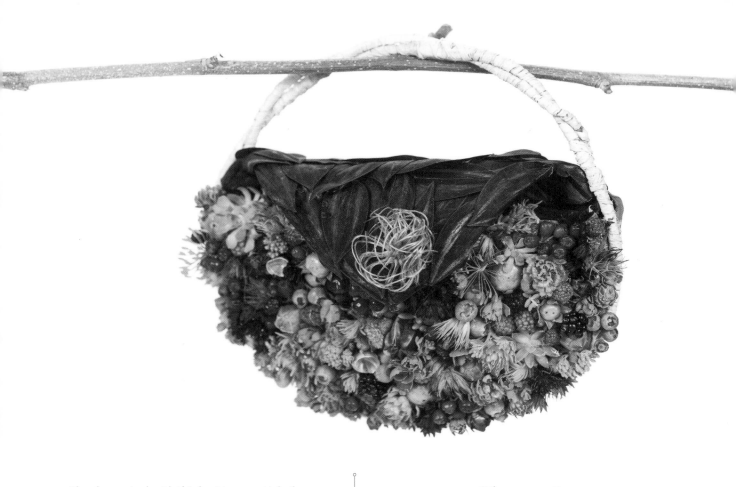

Blends created with this herb's essential oil

Other preparations

_____

COMMON NAME

_____   _____

BOTANICAL NAME   DATE

Parts used   Notes on the plant or harvest

_____   _____
_____   _____
_____   _____
_____   _____

Recipes or medicines created

_____
_____
_____
_____
_____
_____
_____
_____
_____

Blends created with this herb's essential oil

Other preparations

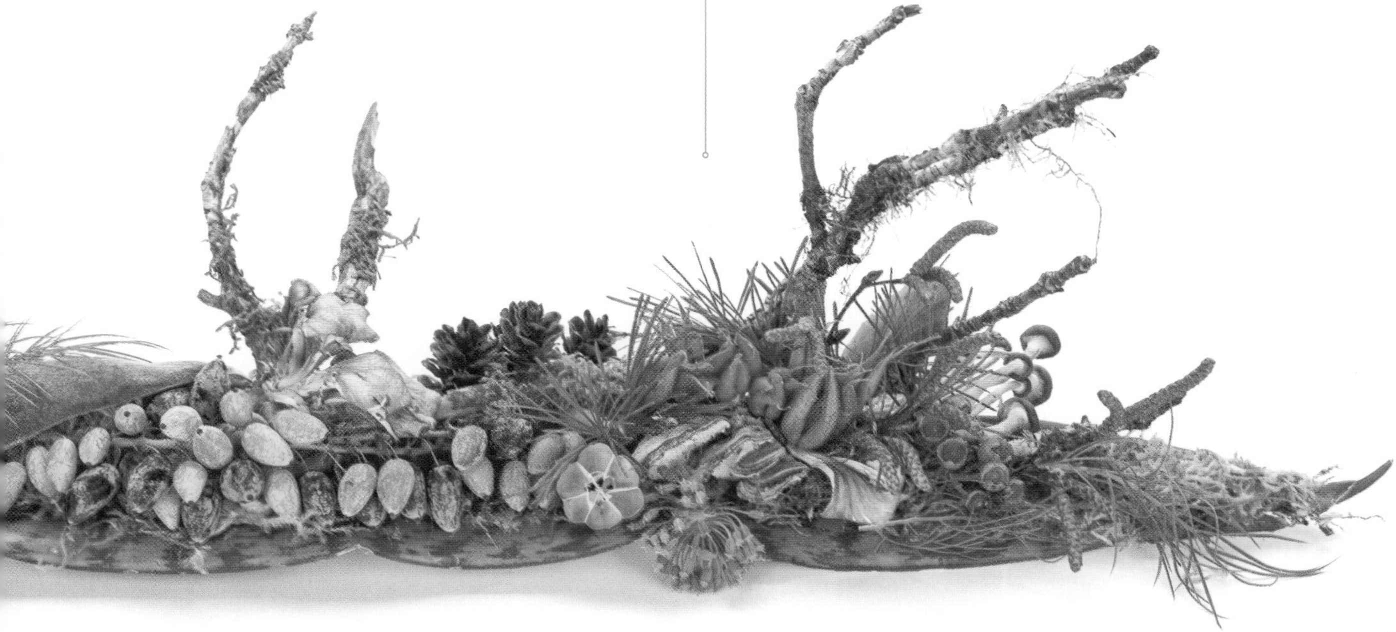

COMMON NAME

BOTANICAL NAME

DATE

Parts used

Notes on the plant or harvest

Recipes or medicines created

Blends created with this herb's essential oil

Other preparations

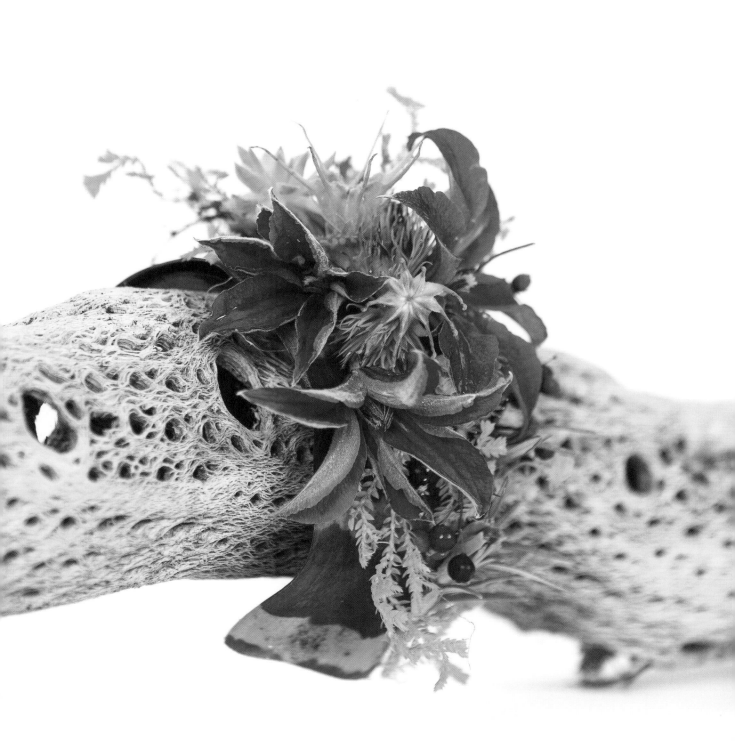

COMMON NAME

DATE

Parts used

Notes on the plant or harvest

Recipes or medicines created

156

Blends created with this herb's essential oil

Other preparations

157

_____

COMMON NAME

_____   _____

BOTANICAL NAME   DATE

Parts used

_____   _____
_____   _____
_____   _____
_____   _____

Notes on the plant or harvest

Recipes or medicines created

_____
_____
_____
_____
_____
_____
_____
_____
_____
_____

Blends created with this herb's essential oil

Other preparations

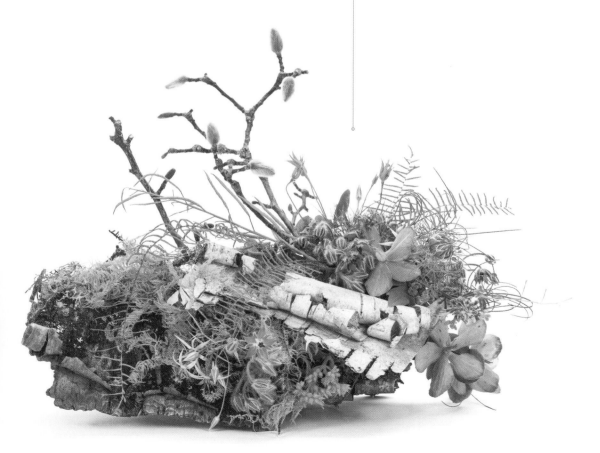

159

COMMON NAME

BOTANICAL NAME

DATE

Parts used

Notes on the plant or harvest

Recipes or medicines created

Blends created with this herb's essential oil

Other preparations

COMMON NAME

BOTANICAL NAME

DATE

Parts used

Notes on the plant or harvest

Recipes or medicines created

Blends created with this herb's essential oil

Other preparations

COMMON NAME

BOTANICAL NAME

DATE

Parts used

Notes on the plant or harvest

Recipes or medicines created

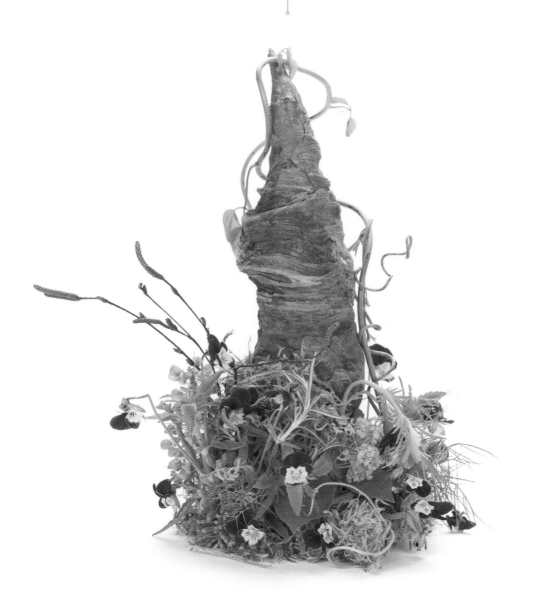

COMMON NAME

BOTANICAL NAME

DATE

⁘ ⟶ ◦o✿o◦ ✿ ◦o✿o◦ ⟵ ⁘

Parts used

Notes on the plant or harvest

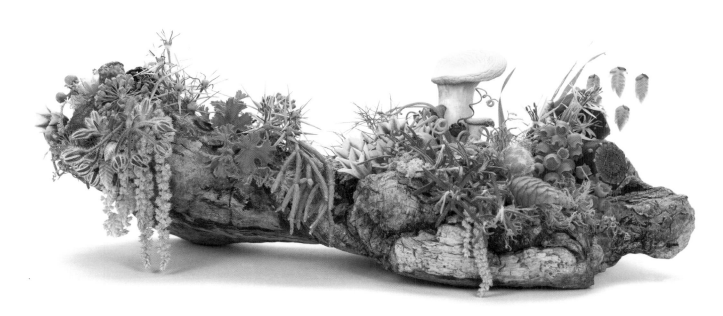

Recipes or medicines created

_____
_____
_____
_____
_____
_____
_____
_____
_____
_____

Blends created with this herb's essential oil

Other preparations

_____

COMMON NAME

_____

BOTANICAL NAME   DATE

Parts used   Notes on the plant or harvest

_____   _____
_____   _____
_____   _____
_____   _____

Recipes or medicines created

_____
_____
_____
_____
_____
_____
_____
_____
_____
_____
_____

Blends created with this herb's essential oil

Other preparations

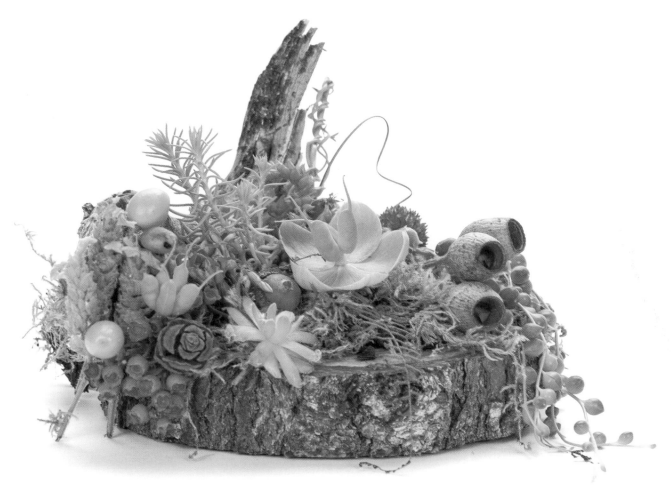

167

_____

COMMON NAME

_____

BOTANICAL NAME   DATE

⚬————————— ❧•❀•❀•☙ —————————⚬

Parts used   Notes on the plant or harvest
⚬————————————⚬   ⚬————————————⚬

_____   _____
_____   _____
_____   _____
_____   _____

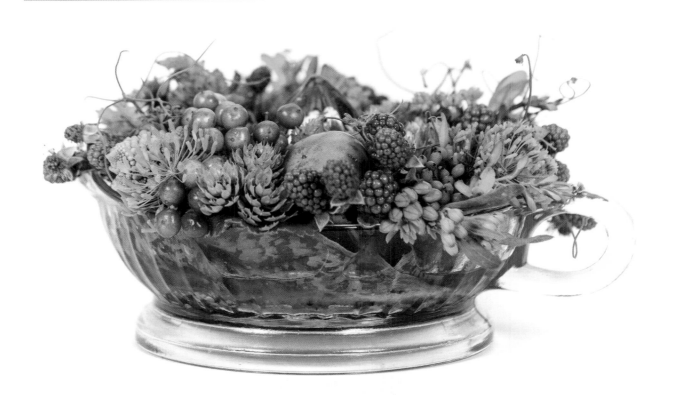

Recipes or medicines created

_____
_____
_____
_____
_____
_____
_____
_____
_____
_____

Blends created with this herb's essential oil

Other preparations

COMMON NAME

BOTANICAL NAME

DATE

Parts used

Notes on the plant or harvest

Recipes or medicines created

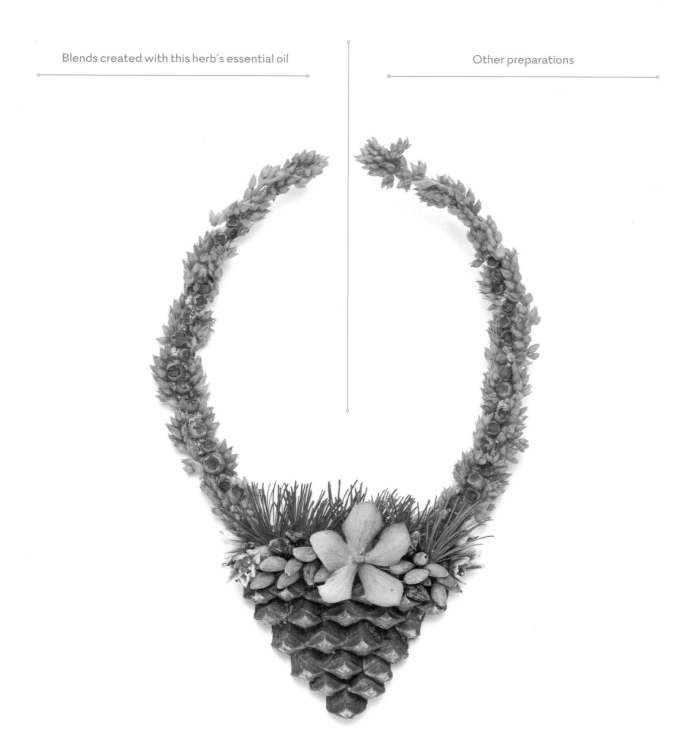

Blends created with this herb's essential oil

Other preparations

COMMON NAME

BOTANICAL NAME

DATE

Parts used

Notes on the plant or harvest

Recipes or medicines created

Blends created with this herb's essential oil

Other preparations

_____

COMMON NAME

_____

BOTANICAL NAME   DATE

— ❧ ❦❧❦❧ ❦❧❦ ❧ —

Parts used

_____
_____
_____
_____

Notes on the plant or harvest

_____
_____
_____
_____

Recipes or medicines created

_____
_____
_____
_____
_____
_____
_____
_____
_____
_____

Blends created with this herb's essential oil

Other preparations

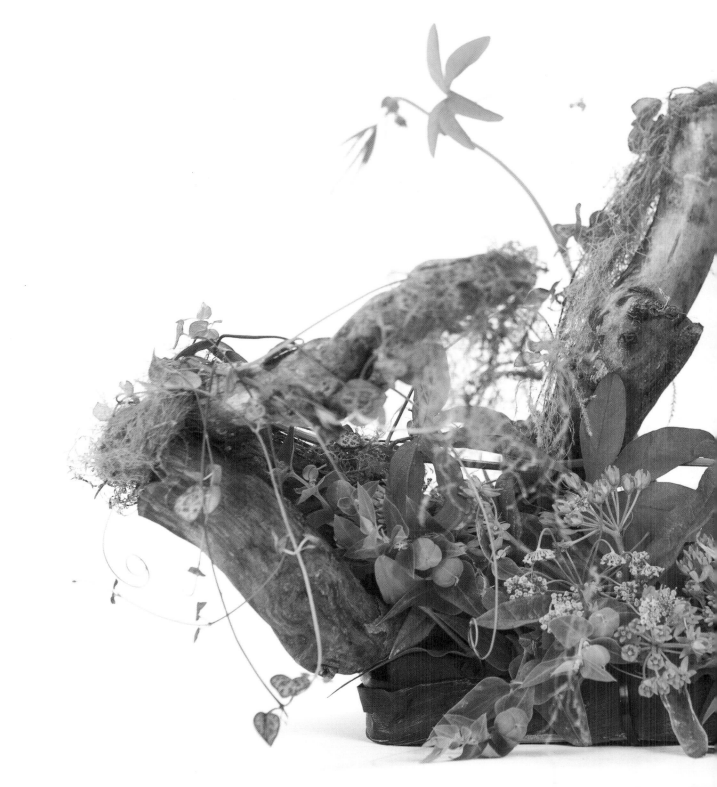

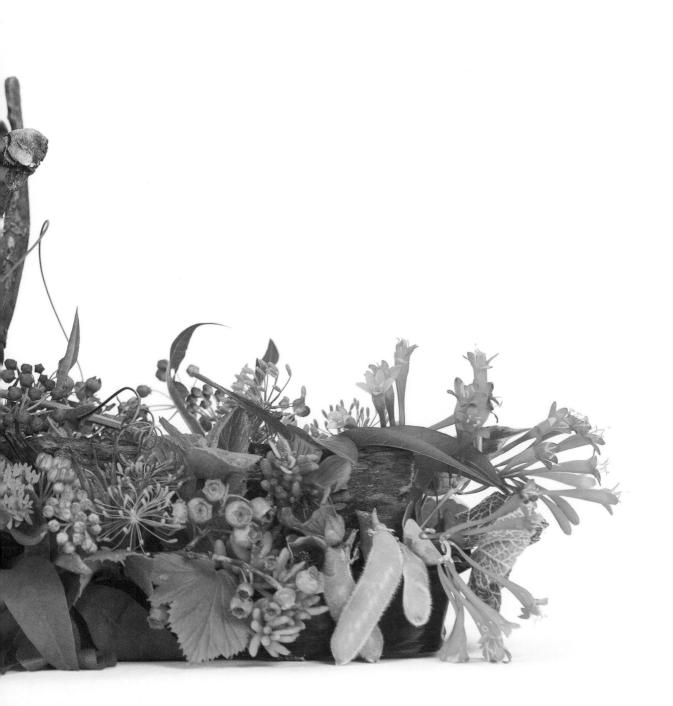

COMMON NAME

BOTANICAL NAME   DATE

Parts used   Notes on the plant or harvest

Recipes or medicines created

Blends created with this herb's essential oil
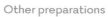

Other preparations

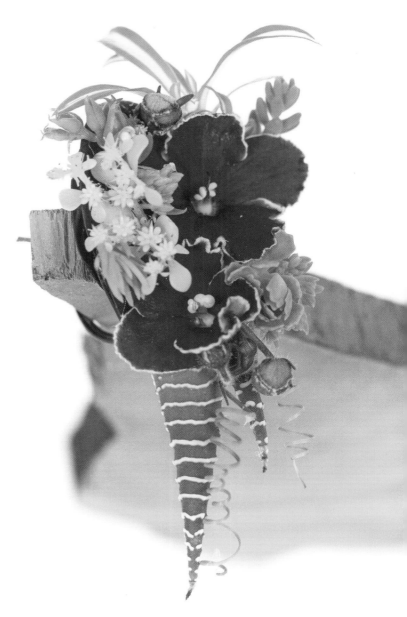

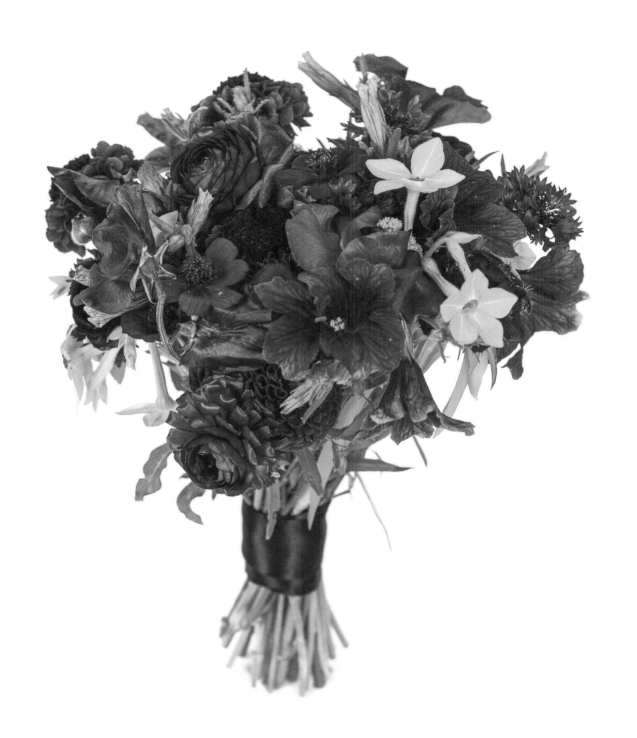

_____

COMMON NAME

_____

BOTANICAL NAME   DATE

———— ❧◦◦❧◦◦❧ ❧◦◦❧ ————

Parts used   Notes on the plant or harvest

_____   _____
_____   _____
_____   _____
_____   _____

Recipes or medicines created   Blends created with this herb's essential oil

_____
_____
_____
_____
_____
_____
_____   Other preparations
_____
_____
_____

_____

COMMON NAME

_____

BOTANICAL NAME   DATE

Parts used

_____
_____
_____
_____

Notes on the plant or harvest

_____
_____
_____
_____

Recipes or medicines created

_____
_____
_____
_____
_____
_____
_____
_____
_____

Blends created with this herb's essential oil

Other preparations

COMMON NAME

_____

BOTANICAL NAME   DATE

Parts used

Notes on the plant or harvest

Recipes or medicines created

Blends created with this herb's essential oil

Other preparations

_____

COMMON NAME

_____   _____

BOTANICAL NAME   DATE

— ❧ ❦ ❧ —

Parts used

_____

_____

_____

_____

Notes on the plant or harvest

_____

_____

_____

_____

Recipes or medicines created

_____

_____

_____

_____

_____

_____

_____

_____

_____

Blends created with this herb's essential oil

Other preparations

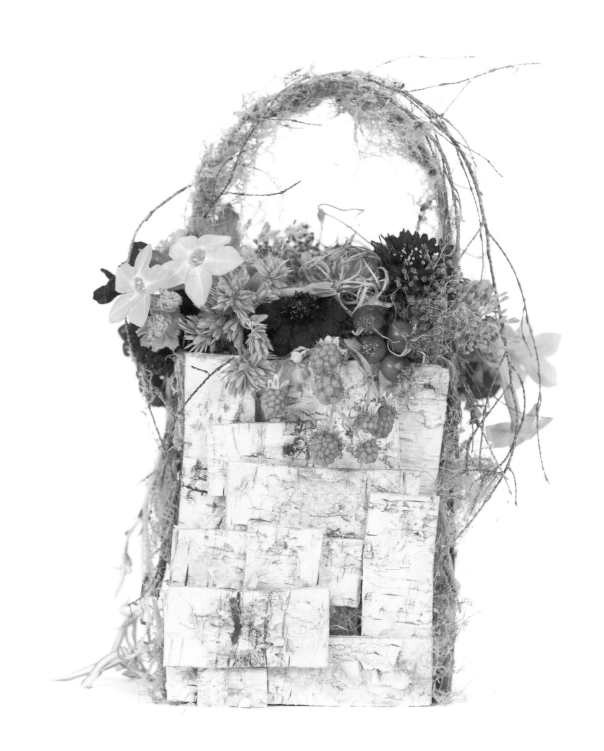

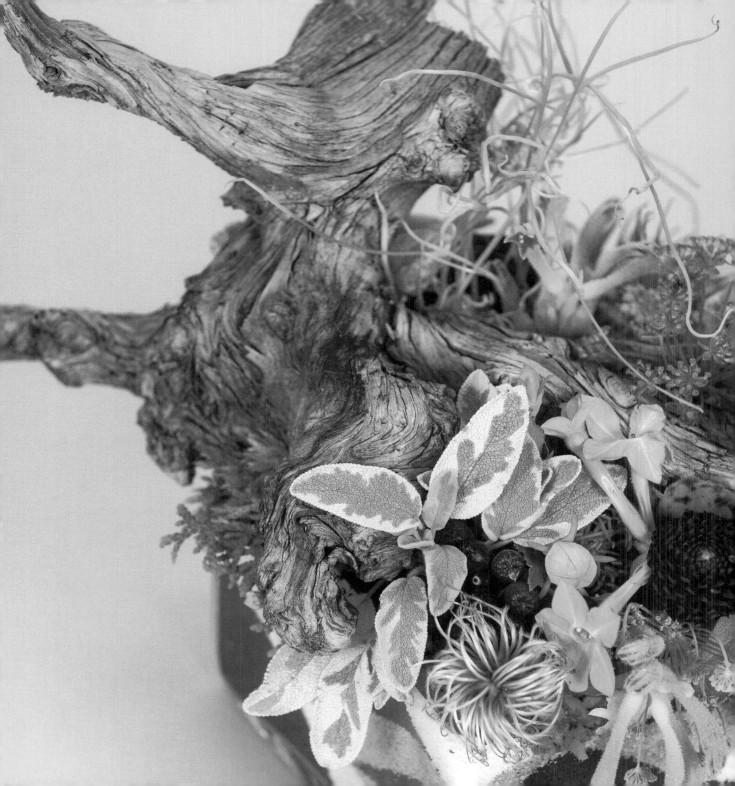

_____

COMMON NAME

_____

BOTANICAL NAME   DATE

———— ·◦◦◦◦◦◦◦· ————

Parts used   Notes on the plant or harvest

_____   _____
_____   _____
_____   _____
_____   _____

Recipes or medicines created   Blends created with this herb's essential oil

_____
_____
_____
_____
_____   Other preparations
_____
_____
_____
_____
_____

BOTANICAL NAME

DATE

Parts used

Notes on the plant or harvest

Recipes or medicines created

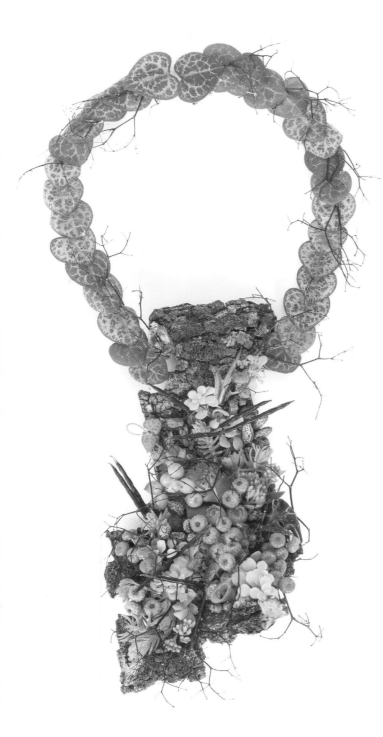

Blends created with this herb's essential oil

Other preparations

187

_____

COMMON NAME

_____   _____

BOTANICAL NAME   DATE

❦ ⸙⸙⸙⸙⸙ ⸙⸙⸙ ⸙

Parts used   Notes on the plant or harvest

_____   _____
_____   _____
_____   _____
_____   _____

Recipes or medicines created

_____
_____
_____
_____
_____
_____
_____
_____
_____
_____

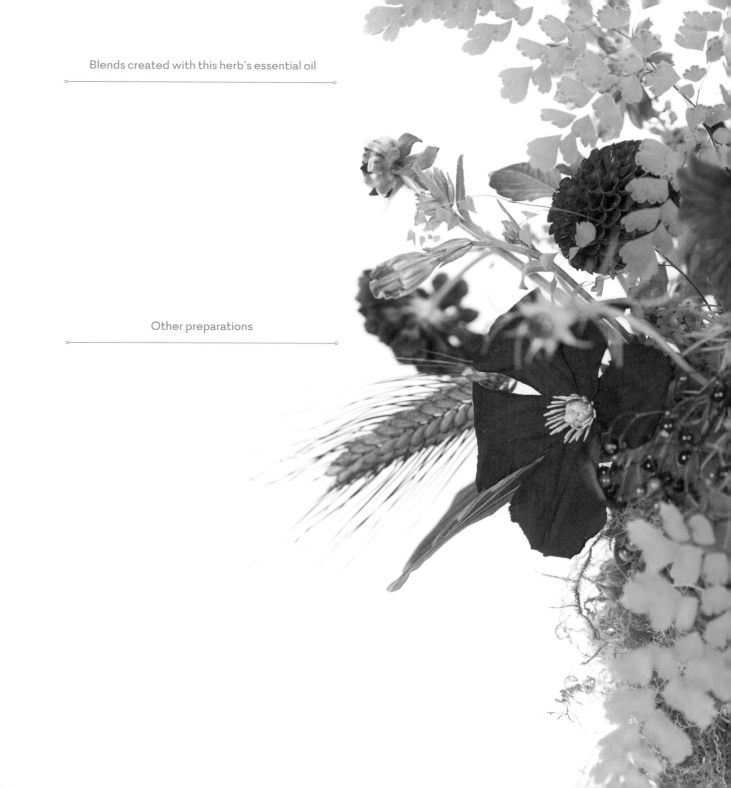

Blends created with this herb's essential oil

Other preparations

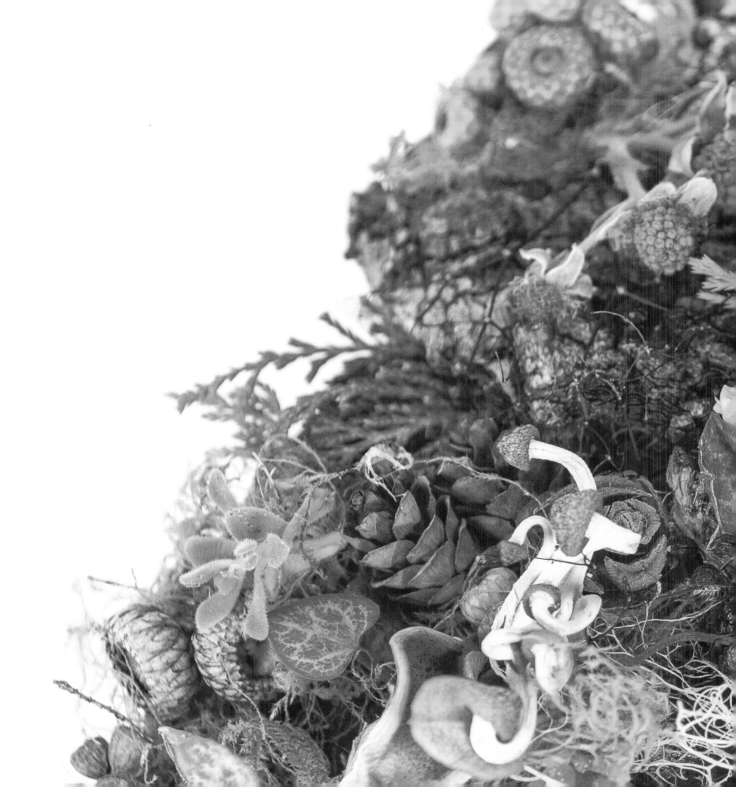

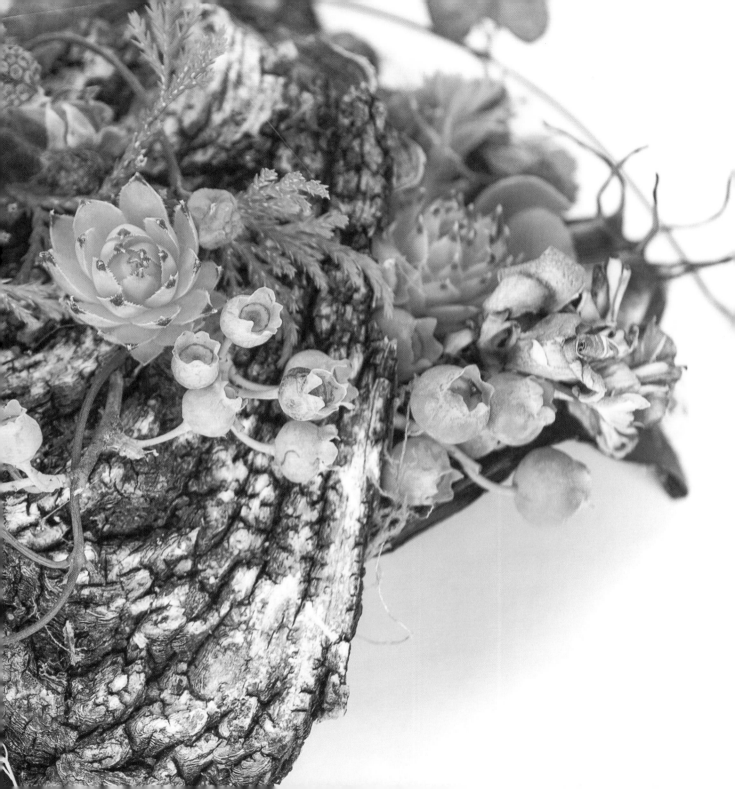

JANUARY

FEBRUARY

Notes from

MARCH

Notes from

APRIL

Notes from

MAY

Notes from
JUNE

Notes from

JULY

AUGUST

OCTOBER

DECEMBER

ARRANGEMENT RECIPES

My deepest appreciation goes to the many local growers and the wholesalers who provided a beautiful selection of seasonal flowers and textures for this project. In particular, I wish to thank Leah Rodgers for letting me peruse her flower farm to handpick an extensive selection of favorites.

I cannot thank photographer Theresa Bear enough for capturing these beautiful images. As a true flower lover, she sees what I see and makes the details simply shine.

Thank you to many friends for their unfailing support, in particular Kate Bryant, Elizabeth Bryant, and Gwen Severson.

Many thanks to Stacee Lawrence and Hillary Caudle at Timber Press for inviting me to collaborate on this project and for giving me all the creative freedom that anyone could dream of. Thanks are due as well to Mia Johnson for designing this lovely volume.

Last but not least, I dedicate this to my late mom, Louise De Wilder, who instilled the love of flowers in me from a very young age. It was a delight to be able to incorporate a design in her first bronzed shoe. Maman, I know you would be proud of me.

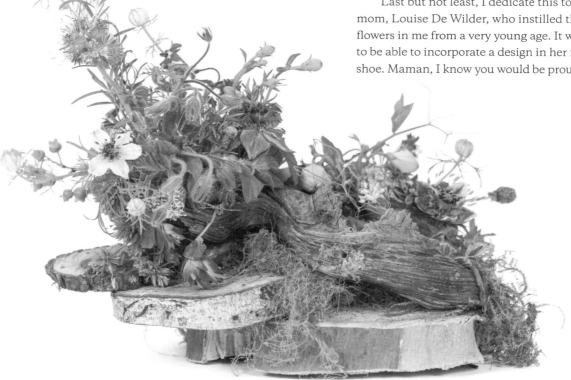

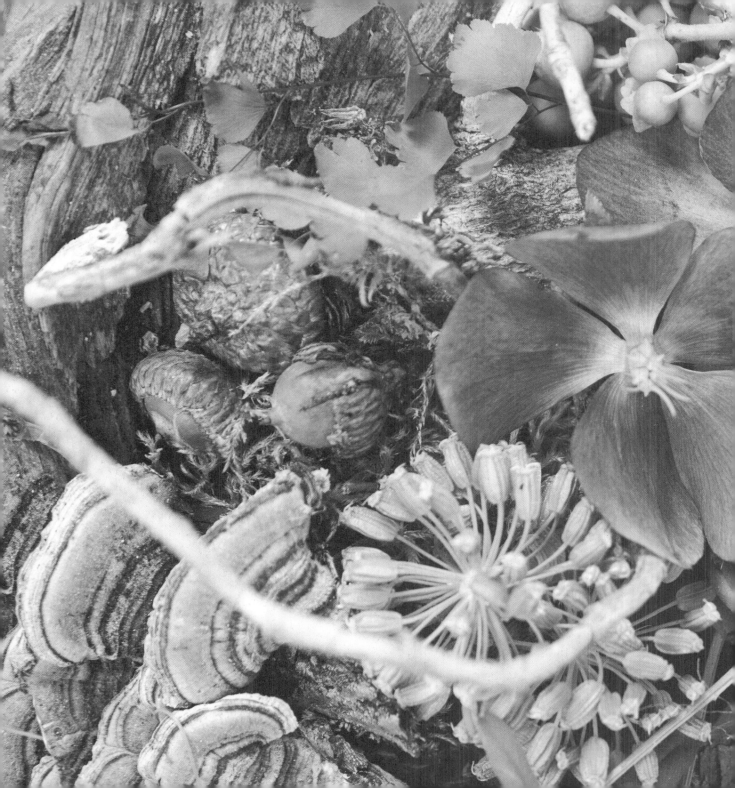